THIN

THROUGH

THE

 POWER

OF

SPIRIT

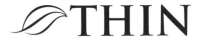

THIN

THROUGH THE

POWER OF

SPIRIT

Creating

Paradise in

Your Weight

and World

Lucia Capodilupo

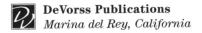

DeVorss Publications
Marina del Rey, California

THIN THROUGH THE POWER OF SPIRIT
© 1999 Lucia Capodilupo
ISBN: 087516-726-8

Library of Congress Catalog Card Number 99-74070
First Edition, 1999

DeVorss & Company
P.O. Box 550
Marina del Rey, CA 90294-0550

Printed in the United States of America

ACKNOWLEDGMENTS

I am grateful to everyone whose support enabled me to bring this book to fruition, especially Julia Holm Azrael, Angela Capodilupo, Arline and Joel Epstein, Jan Gladish, Gary Peattie, Kathleen Thorne-Thomsen, and Arthur Vergara. Additional thanks to Gail Addiss for good advice and to Eileen Mawn for telling me all those years ago that thoughts affect outer reality. I would also like to express my appreciation of everyone who reads this book and is open to the concept of permanent weight loss through spiritual change.

Dedicated to
Rose Schacht, bravest of the brave

in loving memory

CONTENTS

PREFACE

When I was younger, I was very fat. After years of struggling with excess weight, I was lucky enough to realize that I could end this problem once and for all by using spiritual resources. A changed consciousness based on spiritual awareness was my key to liberation.

If you would like to lose weight, you will find in this book a new perspective that can change your weight and transform your way of looking at the world forever. This book will help you move out of the prison of excess weight and into the Paradise-like freedom of a thinner, healthier, and more attractive body. You can be at the weight you desire, and you can begin to get there right now.

Losing weight does not have to be difficult. It becomes simple and natural when you rely on the power of Spirit and allow your higher consciousness to act on your behalf. Relax, and have fun as the process unfolds!

Lucia Capodilupo

1

Making Peace

with the

Physical World

W HY DO WE BECOME FAT? There are many obvious answers, but the root cause of fatness is something deep, subtle, and unrecognized. The root cause of fatness is subconscious unhappiness at the fact of our physical incarnation. This statement represents a new insight into problems of excess weight, and if it sounds strange to you, I hope that you will keep an open mind about it until you finish reading this book. I am sharing this insight with you on the basis of many years of counseling overweight people and my own experience as a formerly fat person.

I am five feet tall, and when I was younger I weighed 205 lb. I lost 95 lb. and have remained at a normal weight for more than 20 years, using this insight and the methods of spiritual change described in this book. I know that you too can lose weight and keep it off if you follow the suggestions given here.

FATNESS AND ALIENATION FROM THE PHYSICAL WORLD

An unwanted weight gain, whether minor or serious, results from feelings of alienation. We tend to put on weight when we are feeling alienated from our work, our mate, our responsibilities, or some other part of the content of our lives. The more serious the feeling of alienation, the more serious our weight problem tends to be. *Obesity results from the most serious type of alienation of all, which is a sense, conscious or unconscious, of alienation from the physical world itself.*

We are spiritual beings who came to Earth and took on bodies in order to assist in the perfecting of the world. Unfortunately, this original purpose of our incarnation in the physical world has been forgotten by most of us. When we forget our purpose in taking physical form, life on the physical plane can seem pointless, burdensome, and restrictive. We feel alienated from the physical world and subconsciously long for the unbounded state of our earlier, nonphysical existence.

Time and again, people I have counseled who are extremely heavy have directly and indirectly revealed that they are unhappy at being here in the physical world and that they long to be somewhere else. This is especially true of those obese people I know who have strong spiritual yearnings. Our spirituality, or desire for greater experience of the Divine, should be our greatest asset in making our bodies healthy and free of weight problems; instead, we often misdirect our spirituality into a longing to "escape" from the physical world.

FATNESS AND ANOREXIA

When we have a negative attitude towards physical existence, many physical problems can arise. In recent decades, we have seen the unhappy result of our subconscious desire to be nonphysical in the development of anorexia and other body-diminishing disorders among teenage girls. Fatness is the opposite side of anorexia on the dangerous coin of aversion to the physical world. Fatness and anorexia each occur because in our alienation from the physical world we subconsciously view the physical world as evil.

Anorexia results when we subconsciously feel so ashamed of our physicality that we want to shrink from sight. Fatness results when we subconsciously feel so oppressed by our physicality that we view the body as the prison of the soul. When the metaphor of the body as the prison of the soul becomes the governing metaphor of our lives, this metaphor becomes internalized in the body itself. Subconsciously ruled by this metaphor, we produce a body that really does imprison us behind a wall of fat.

If we wish to free ourselves from excess weight once and for all, our negative philosophy, or way of looking at the world and our purpose in it, must change. This book offers an approach to weight loss that utilizes spiritual resources to help you change your philosophy, your psychology, your body image, and your food choices. The place to begin is with your philosophy, since *the way you view the world and the purpose of physical existence is the predominant factor in excess weight.* The other causes of excess weight are much easier to overcome once the root cause of unhappiness at the fact of physical existence is dealt with.

In this chapter we will discuss our new insight in depth. We will focus on accepting the physical world as good and understanding that the purpose of physical incarnation is to help perfect the world—or, as I like to phrase it, to create Paradise on Earth. Making this radical shift in your subconscious view of the world and perception of the purpose of physical existence can set you free from the cycle of compulsive eating and obsessing about food. You can dissolve your old weight pattern by dissolving your misconceptions about physicality. You can attain your perfect weight by making peace with the physical world.

✐ PERFECT WEIGHT

Ideas about weight are highly relative, and concepts of how much weight is attractive vary widely from culture to culture. By "perfect weight" I am *not* talking about the impossible standards of thinness dictated by the media and the fashion industry, nor the tortured concept of perfection that has contributed to so much anorexia and bulimia. By "perfect weight" I *am* talking about the weight that is perfect for your good health, radiance, and fitness, given your height and bone structure.

If you have been both slender and fat, you probably can remember what your perfect weight felt like. Perfect weight is the weight at which your body performs its best, and your life is free from preoccupation with weight and obsession with eating. Perfect weight is your body's natural state. It provides your body with maximum freedom of activity and your mind with minimum self-distraction. Perfect weight is your birthright, and it should be a given for everyone, so that no one has to waste energy on weight-related problems and predicaments.

Modern industrial cultures, influenced by the media's obsession with thinness, tend to look down on fat people and marginalize them, while at the same time expanding the definition of *fat* so that more and more people are viewed as unacceptably overweight. Even Marilyn Monroe, whose figure was considered perfect in the late 1950s and early 1960s, would be judged too heavy by today's standards. In many traditional cultures, on the other hand, having more weight rather than less is viewed as an asset, and in many cases fatness is regarded as beautiful in its own right.

CULTURAL ATTITUDES

This difference in cultural attitudes was brought home to me in a very personal way when I went on a summer study tour in the Soviet Union in the late 1960s to learn the Russian language. At the time I weighed 190 lb.—less than my all-time high of 205, but still a hefty amount for someone only 5' tall. As part of the study tour, our American student group spent some time in the Republic of Azerbaijan, in Baku, a city which in the late '60s retained many traditional Near Eastern values despite 50 years of Soviet government. To my surprise, in Baku I was regarded as a great beauty because of my weight. "How fat and beautiful you are!" a local Communist Party official admiringly whispered in my ear at one of the compulsory "friendship" evenings held for foreign visitors. "You could be the wife of a khan!"

"You're lucky that we have Soviet power in Azerbaijan now, " another official told me one day. "In the old days, a beautiful fat girl like you would have been carried off into the hills by bandits and given to their chief."

Everywhere I went, I was the center of admiring attention. When I went out to restaurants in the evening with other students, men sitting at adjacent tables would invariably send champagne and grapes to our table in my honor and drink toasts to me from across the room. After word about this spread, my fellow students would vie with each other to get to sit at my table. In the mornings I would find anonymous gifts of melon, grapes, and wine left outside my hotel room door in tribute to my beauty. What a difference from life in America! For the first time it struck me that being beautiful was not so much a question of *how you looked* as of *where you were*.

Fat is still considered very beautiful in many areas of the world. Recently I had a part-time job in a shop whose staff came from a number of different countries. The shop was located in a section of Manhattan frequented by many actors, actresses, and models, and some extremely beautiful and successful African-American models were among our regular customers. While the American staff members would often comment on how striking these models were, the staff members from Senegal, on the other hand, expressed sorrow for these same young women! It was a shame, they said, that such nice young women were so thin; in Senegal no one would ever find them attractive.

NO ABSOLUTE STANDARDS

Thus there are no absolute standards for weight, and we should take the standards of our own thinness-obsessed culture with more than just a grain of salt. It is not a crime to be fat, and we are not bad people for being fat. If we want to lose weight, it is best to start from a position of self-acceptance, knowing that value judgments about fat are entirely relative and that the perfect weight for a particular body is the weight at which that body experiences maximum ease and health, regardless of the artificial standards dictated by the media and the fashion industry. Each body has its own innate standard, determined by its bone structure and height.

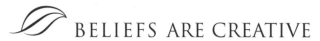 BELIEFS ARE CREATIVE

To achieve the weight that is perfect for your body, you must change your attitude of alienation from the physical world. Alienation results not only from having forgotten our reason for incarnating but also from the dualistic philosophy that has arisen from our forgetting. Dualistic thinking has pervaded our civilization for centuries and has generated strong subconscious hatred of the physical world. In dualistic thinking, matter and spirit are seen not as the continuum of a single unity but rather as forces separate from and diametrically opposed to each other. Dualistic thinking has led many people to the mistaken subconscious conclusion that since spirituality is good, physicality must be evil.

Your body, it goes without saying, is made of physical matter. If you believe that the physical world is evil, you will automatically perceive your body as evil. If you view the physical world as being in opposition to higher spiritual pursuits, you will view physical existence as oppressive, and the body as the prison of the soul. Your attitude towards the body can be nothing but negative if you adhere to a dualistic philosophy of matter and spirit.

OUR BELIEFS CREATE OUR EXPERIENCES

The fact that you may be unaware of holding negative beliefs about the physical world and the body unfortunately will not protect you from the harmful impact of holding these beliefs in your subconscious mind. The thought patterns that dominate our mind invariably out-picture as our experience. Our experiences reflect our beliefs; to be more precise, our innermost beliefs create our experiences, or outer reality, as surely as a command. Whether we have bodies that are overweight, under-weight, or perfect weight depends on the belief that is cre-ating or "programming" our weight experience. Persistent excess weight and obesity result when we believe that the physical world and the body are evil, and that the body is the prison of the soul. Our negative attitude towards phys-icality and the body inevitably impels us to create a body that is weighed down and imprisoned by fat.

It is ironic that many of us currently and formerly fat people have been viewed as self-indulgent sensualists by others, when actually our excessive eating was programmed by our subconscious aversion to the physical world.

Some people find it hard to accept that our beliefs cre-ate our outer reality. If you have resistance to this idea, I ask you to keep an open mind about it and accept it as a working premise. You will see for yourself what happens if you accept this idea and change to more positive beliefs about the physical world and the body.

I am using the word *beliefs* here to encompass not only beliefs but also all the emotions, thoughts, judgments, commentaries, attitudes, and expectations that make up the inner world of our conscious and subconscious minds. All of these mental/emotional components act upon the stuff of the universe to produce all of our experiences. This happens constantly, and in every aspect of our lives, from the most mundane to the most sublime; it is a fun-damental law of the universe that our external conditions are generated in keeping with our "beliefs," both individ-ual and societal.

Eastern religions have long taught the correlation of outer conditions with inner states. Jesus also said that it is done unto us according to our belief. He was referring not simply to the need to have faith if we wish to experience miracles, but also to the law that all our experiences result from our system of beliefs. This basic law of the universe that Jesus was describing is the law of karma.

Karma has been popularly understood to mean that every action has a consequence, and this is correct as far as it goes. However, the deeper meaning of karma is that inner conditions have outer consequences. St. Paul was well aware of this when he urged the early Christians to think on "whatsoever things are true, noble, right, pure, lovely, and honorable." Like many other spiritual teachers, Paul realized that peaceful thoughts produce harmonious outer conditions.

MONITORING OUR BELIEFS

It's important that we monitor our beliefs, since they are so very creative. Sometimes we can easily see the relationship between inner beliefs and outer experience. For example, almost everyone has had the experience of riding with a friend who finds a parking space where it's almost impossible to find one, and who says, "I knew I'd find a space" or "I always get a space when I come here." Belief manifests as experience all the time, though it may not always be so directly observable as in the primitive example above.

What happens is that our beliefs create a general climate or "vibration" that attracts experiences with a similar "vibration" to us. Everyone, for instance, has observed that when we are upset, we tend to have additional upsetting experiences. We have all had those weeks in which we receive bad news and then our car has a flat tire, our hot water heater breaks down, and things continue to go wrong until some level of equilibrium is restored. We have also had periods in which good happenings were consistently followed by even better ones. *We tend to get more of whatever is dominating our consciousness.*

MASS BELIEFS

Our external reality will be positive or negative depending on our individual and mass consciousness, or the clusters of mental/emotional perception we are holding about various aspects of life. Mass beliefs are especially potent and create vibrations that can affect us even when we would never personally subscribe to these beliefs. The implications for this on the societal level are vast. Our negative mass beliefs, emotions, and other inner postures have produced vibrations conducive to war, illness, poverty, loneliness, crime, failure, and other forms of suffering. None of these problems is necessary; all are eradicable once we really accept the law of "inner produces outer."

While it may take society a while to accept this law, more and more individuals are becoming aware of it and are using it to improve their lives. According to this law, if you want your weight to change, you must change internally. As Emily Dickinson wrote in another context, "the Outer from the Inner/derives its Magnitude".

The law of "inner produces outer" is impersonal, not punitive, and provides an avenue of hope and renewal. The law is especially easy to apply to weight loss, since your weight depends so completely on you. You do not have to use the law to change anyone's thinking but your own. Once you learn to work the law to your advantage, it will mean your liberation from excess weight forever.

BECOMING AWARE OF WHAT YOU REALLY THINK

To use the law to your advantage, you must become aware of what your negative beliefs and feelings really are and then change them so that your inner state will be in keeping with the outer state you desire. We usually assume that we know what we really believe, think, or feel about a subject; however, our subconscious attitudes towards this subject may vary greatly from our conscious ones, and it is our subconscious ones that affect us. For instance, a person may consciously want financial security yet may always wind up in financial difficulties because she subconsciously believes that it's wrong to have money, or that she's incapable of making money. Her subconscious belief is operating to always keep her in a state of financial lack, despite her conscious efforts to acquire money.

If your outer experiences aren't in keeping with what you want, know that something in your inner state is preventing it. There is no blame involved here. Subconsciously affected as we all have been by mass beliefs and by our past experiences of this and other lifetimes, our inner state is in many ways beyond our conscious control. The more aware we can become of our inner state, however, the more we can consciously change it.

CHARACTER PARTS

Our inner state is often governed by certain negative aspects of our personality that are usually dormant but that can come to the fore whether we consciously want them to or not. These usually submerged parts of our character (or *Character Parts,* as I like to call them) often have completely different beliefs, needs and agendas from our conscious selves and rule us at a subconscious level.

Everyone has Character Parts. In my case, I most easily recognize the Brat ("I'm not going to do this, and nobody can make me"), the Rebellious Teenager ("Don't tell me what to do!"), the hypercritical Hanging Judge ("Why do people get on the bus when they don't have the right change handy? They should be thrown off!"), and a spaced-out indolent part that I call Madame Oblomova, named after the languid title character in the Russian novel Oblomov who spends a good part of the day lounging around in his dressing gown ("It's 4:00 P.M. already, and I don't have a clue where the day has gone."). I also have a Character Part that I call the Devouring Monster ("I'm upset and I'm going to eat everything up.").

These parts of me are often completely at odds with my conscious self, but they do exist, and I am getting better at recognizing when they are motivating me and when I am experiencing emotions connected with them and not my more rational part. You can become more aware of your inner state by examining your reactions and behavior to see if they are consistent with your conscious self or instead reflect the influence of your Character Parts. The more aware you become of when a Character Part is dominating you, the easier it will be to transcend its influence.

FEEDBACK

You can also become aware of the contents of your inner life by accepting your external reality as feedback about your inner state. For example, if you constantly wind up with an antagonistic boss, take this as feedback that you are holding negative beliefs about authority or about your relationship to authority. If the people you are romantically involved with always turn out to be emotional deadbeats, take this as feedback that you hold negative beliefs about the opposite sex or about love relationships.

The body, of course, is the original feedback device! We give it food, and the weight and shape it acquires allow us to monitor and change the deep inner beliefs that are affecting our food intake and weight production. If you are consistently overweight, you are being given feedback that a negative core attitude dominates your thinking about the body; the heavier the excess weight, the more extreme the negativity.

HATRED OF THE PHYSICAL BODY

Using the state of your body as feedback, you can see that if you are overweight or obese, there must be an element of body hatred at work in your psyche. Why would you burden your body with excess poundage to carry around if you didn't hate it? Why would you endanger its health and restrict its options for love, admiration, and physical activity of all kinds? You must renounce body hatred and change your attitude towards your body if you want to reach your perfect weight.

Hatred of the body comes from the hidden belief that the physical world is evil. Your body is the place where you indwell the physical world most immediately; it is the point at which your personality intersects the physical world. Your body, is moreover, a microcosm of the larger physical world. There is no way that you can separate your attitude toward your body from your attitude towards the physical world in general.

There can be no body hatred without hatred of the physical world, and no body love without love of the physical world. Your attitude towards the physical world is the prime indicator of whether or not you will experience excess weight. The stronger your belief, conscious or unconscious, that the physical world is evil, the more you will hate your body, and the more excess weight you will manifest. *Obese people are suffering from an extreme subconscious revulsion towards the physical world, which they perceive as an evil place full of danger, misery, dirt, and disappointment.*

The belief that physical matter is evil has a long history in our Western civilization, going back to Zoroastrianism, Manichaeism, Gnosticism, and other ancient teachings that posited two opposing creative principles in the universe, one good and one evil. In these systems, matter was seen as derived from the evil principle. In the Middle Ages, popular heretical Christian groups who were influenced by these traditions, such as the Bogomils in the Balkans and the Cathars in the South of France, actively taught that the body was created by the Devil.

The official teaching of the Catholic Church always upheld the goodness of the created universe, including the body, but in fact many Church representatives shared the anti-somatic prejudices of other traditions. Moreover, the Church was heavily influenced by the Platonic concept that the body and the soul, matter and non-matter, are in opposition, and that the body is the prison of the soul.

Despite its official belief in the goodness of the physical world and the human body, the Church in practice commonly preached a world view that saw the physical world as a valley of tears and the human body as a cesspool of evil and corruption. This negative view, which is inconsistent with the Church's own teaching, has persisted throughout the history of Western Christianity, and in Catholic circles has waned only in recent decades. The Eastern Church fortunately espoused an attitude more in keeping with the love of the body implicit in Christ's resurrection.

"THE WORLD, THE FLESH, AND THE DEVIL"

Prejudice against the body among the clergy has certainly not been restricted to Catholics. You can turn to Christian moralism of almost any denomination and time period, and whether you are considering such diverse preachers as the medieval Catholic saint Bernard of Clairvaux, the Puritan Jonathan Edwards, or contemporary revivalists on Sunday radio programs, you will find the body consistently represented as evil. The familiar expression "the world, the flesh, and the devil," used to describe the sources of human temptation, indirectly associates the physical world and the body with the diabolical.

If you were raised in a Western country, you can have a subconscious anti-somatic prejudice even if you never were exposed to negative preaching about the body and

never heard of Gnosticism or Manichaeism. As a participant in our Western society, you share in its collective
unconscious, which has been deeply imbued with body
hatred and disgust at the physical world. If you are a "spiritual" person raised in this culture, you are especially
prone to this negative view of physical reality.

Most people are completely unaware of the fact that
they subconsciously see the physical world, and therefore
their bodies, as evil. If you don't believe that you hold a
negative view of physical reality, ask yourself what your
immediate reaction is to the phrase, "It's a wonderful
world." If your immediate response is "Oh, yeah? What
about all the poverty, crime, suffering, earthquakes, etc.?"
you can see that you are operating from the position that
the world is evil. This negative view must be changed if
you want to achieve your perfect weight once and for all.

UNDERSTANDING THE PURPOSE OF PHYSICAL INCARNATION

The belief that the physical world is evil, and the dualistic
concept that the physical world is evil whereas the spiritual world is good, come not only from forgetting our true
purpose in incarnating but also from erroneously attributing a false purpose to our entry into the physical plane.
Having forgotten that our purpose is to perfect the world,
many souls come to earth with the mistaken belief that the
point of our sojourn is to purify or develop ourselves by
suffering. If you believe that the purpose of our physical
life is to suffer, then it makes sense to believe that the
physical world and the body are evil.

However, we are not here to suffer, and physical incarnation is not meant to be a punishment. We come to the
physical realm in order to perfect it by our expression of

Divine qualities and to enjoy ourselves in the process. We come to create Paradise on Earth.

CREATING PARADISE ON EARTH

By Paradise on Earth I mean a state reflective of all the wonderful conditions we usually associate with Paradise, such as joy, love, abundance, sharing, an end to suffering, and most of all a deep sense of union with the Divine and with other souls.

Creating Paradise on Earth is not a new idea. Judaism has the concept of *"tikkun,"* or "repairing" the world, in which humankind cooperates with the Creator in perfecting the world. In Christianity, it is incumbent on Christians to participate in the Holy Spirit's work of sanctifying and perfecting the world. Focus on such participation has been particularly strong in Eastern Orthodox Christianity, which emphasizes Christ's redemption not just of humankind but of the whole world. But all Christians invoke Paradise on Earth when praying "Thy kingdom come, Thy will be done on Earth as it is in Heaven."

To create Paradise on Earth is our mission. It is also the deepest desire of our Higher Self.

OUR HIGHER SELF

We each have a Higher Self (sometimes called our Soul Nature or spirit) which is that aspect of ourselves "made in the image and likeness" of our Creator and most directly infused with the Divine. I believe that the Higher Self is a spiritual energy that exists in many different energy realms at the same time and that enjoys expressing the Divine throughout these realms. The physical world is an energy realm; modern physics has documented that physical matter is simply energy slowed down to a vibration that gives it an appearance of solidity. As an energy realm, the physical world is one of the natural playgrounds of the Higher Self and a natural medium for its expression of Divine Perfection.

It's crucial that we stop operating from the level of our personality, or our everyday self, and start taking into account the needs and purposes of our Higher Self. Some people are not even aware that they have a Soul Nature or Higher Self. Other people realize that they have one, yet refuse to allow this realization to influence their lives in any way. If we want our lives to be meaningful, we must become aware of the Higher Self's nature and desires and make its priorities our own.

EXPRESSING THE DIVINE

The Higher Self is totally imbued with the Divine. It is therefore unbounded, blissful, joyous, harmonious, loving, creative, and perfect. Like our Creator, from whom it emanates, the Higher Self is an artist whose nature it is to express Divine Perfection through its creations. These creations include the many wonderful works that the Higher Self wishes to manifest on the physical plane and that would make Earth like Paradise.

The artistic nature of the Divine, and the strength of the artistic impulse inherent within the Higher Self, cannot be emphasized enough. It is this primal artistic impulse of the Higher Self that is paramount in its decision to enter the physical plane and take on a physical body. It was in order to create, artist-like, experiences of beauty, goodness, and harmony that we came to Earth in the first place.

It's important that we actively remember this original purpose of ours. Only by doing so can we free ourselves from believing that the physical world and the body are evil and that we are here to suffer. Only by remembering can we liberate ourselves from the harmful impact our mistaken beliefs have had on our external reality.

Your Higher Self is multidimensional and exists on many planes simultaneously. It exists on the physical plane through you in your present and your other physical reincarnations. At the same time, it exists in a host of nonphysical realms, where it experiences the many different aspects of existence appropriate to these realms.

LIMITATIONS OF THE PHYSICAL REALM

The physical realm has many obvious limitations compared to the nonmaterial realms. In the physical world, you are dependent on your body for knowledge and for activity, and you are limited by your body's sensory and expressive capabilities as well as by forces such as the law of gravity. Moreover, in the physical realm you are subject to the barriers of time, through which we experience day and night, the seasons, and all the events of our lives and history in a sequential fashion, rather than experiencing them simultaneously or with the flexibility to move freely between past, present, and future. Despite these many limitations, the Higher Self freely chooses to enter the physical plane.

Why does the unbounded Soul or Higher Self voluntarily subject itself to the limitations of the physical world? It does so for the artistic satisfaction of working within a confined medium to create expressions of Divine Perfection. The limitations of the physical world are a joyous challenge to the artistic nature of the Higher Self.

HIGHER SELF WELCOMES THE CHALLENGE

Working within self-set limits is a challenge frequently chosen by artists. There is a wonderful sonnet by Wordsworth, about the pleasures of sonnet-writing, in which he expresses the poet's satisfaction in working within the restrictive medium of the sonnet form. In this sonnet, titled "Nuns Fret Not at Their Convent's Narrow Room," Wordsworth compares the contentment of the artist who chooses to work within a confined medium to the contentment of nuns, hermits, students, and others who carry out their life work within voluntarily chosen constraints.

Wordsworth writes: "Nuns fret not at their convent's narrow room;/And hermits are contented with their cells;/And students with their pensive citadels;/Maids at the wheel, the weaver at his loom,/Sit blithe and happy; . . . In truth, the prison, into which we doom/Ourselves, no prison is . . ."

The physical world (and the body in particular) is similarly not a prison, despite what certain philosophers and clergy have declared over the centuries. The Higher Self chooses to take on the restrictions of physical incarnation just as the sonnet-writer in Wordsworth's sonnet chooses to take on the restrictions of the sonnet form. Both the Higher Self and the sonnet-writer are artists intent on working within finite but highly focused forms. Both enjoy the challenge and the opportunity for focus which self-imposed limitations present to their creative genius.

You can love the physical world because it is your freely chosen medium. If your body has been functioning as a prison, it is because you have viewed physical matter as a prison rather than as an artistic medium for creating wonderful works of body, life, and environment. There is nothing intrinsically bad about physicality, any more than any other artistic medium, such as painting, sculpture, or music could be considered intrinsically bad. It is time to release your beliefs that the body is evil and the physical world is meant for suffering, and cooperate with your Higher Self's goal of creatively expressing Divine Perfection on the physical plane.

YOUR PHYSICAL BODY AND THE BODY OF PLANET EARTH

Because we've believed in various ways, consciously and subconsciously, that physicality is evil, we've been locked into deep, subconscious hatred of the physical world. This hatred has dire repercussions not just for our bodies but for the life of Planet Earth as well.

Like the body, Planet Earth is a visible, tangible, accessible microcosm of the macrocosm that is the entire physical universe. Our subconscious feelings about the physical plane are reflected in our attitude towards Planet Earth as well as towards the body. For those of us raised in the West, our identification of the body with Planet Earth is especially strong, since in the Bible Adam is created out of earth. Christian traditional burial stresses the identity of *body* with *earth;* the point is made that the body is being returned to the earth whence it came, "ashes to ashes, dust to dust." At very basic levels of our consciousness, the Earth and body are interchangeable symbols. As a society, we tend to subconsciously view the Earth the way we view our bodies—that is, unfortunately, as evil. *Our subconscious body hatred is paralleled by a deep subconscious hatred of Planet Earth.*

As our bodies, so the Earth

If this seems far-fetched, one has only to stop and reflect on our parallel treatment of our bodies and Planet Earth. It is not just coincidence that we have an epidemic of excess weight and obesity in our society at the same time that our Earth is suffering so severely from an epidemic of garbage dumping, rubbish accumulation, industrial pollution, oil spills, and nuclear contamination. We are behaving towards the Earth as we behave towards our

bodies, trashing the Earth with excess waste and toxins as
we trash our bodies with excessive and detrimental food.
We are punishing the Earth as we punish the body, bur-
dening it with junk overload, disturbing its intrinsic harmony, and destroying its natural beauty. We are turning
the physical world, which was supposed to be our artistic
medium, into a moribund environment increasingly incapable of sustaining life. Why should we treat our bodies
and the Earth like this? Why would we act this way, if not
from often unconscious, unresolved hatred?

Our affluence has permitted us to express our subconscious hatred of the physical world to an extent never
before possible. Obesity and the massive pollution of the
Earth can only occur in conditions of affluence; societies
that do not have enough to eat cannot burden their bodies
with fat or destroy their environment with garbage. We
who live in wealthy societies have ventured on a course of
self-destruction that is incomprehensible on the surface
but that makes sense if we realize that we are motivated
by hatred of the body, and by extension, Planet Earth.

ACCEPTING AND LOVING OUR PHYSICALITY

It's time to stop now. The stakes are too high to continue
in our negative thinking. We must change our consciousness about the body at the very deepest level, giving up
body hatred for body love. Our treatment of Planet Earth
cannot change until we start viewing the body, and the
physical plane in general, as good. We must make a conscious decision to accept the physical world as good and
thus come to love the fact of our physicality. When we
truly perceive the physical world as good, we will have no
need to punish our planet by environmental abuse or our
bodies by becoming fat.

✎ RESOLVING TO CHANGE YOUR PHILOSOPHY

If your deeply held belief that the physical world and the body are evil does not change, your weight-loss efforts will not succeed. You will remain trapped in a subconscious body hatred that impels you to persist in punishing your body with fat. Changing your philosophy is essential, and you can start this change in world view now.

First, acknowledge that you do have a subconscious belief in the evilness of the physical world and the body. *Secondly,* apologize to your Higher Self and to your Creator for having gotten off track and fallen into this belief. *Third,* state your intention to change your negative belief to a belief that the world and the body are good.

You can do this right now, before proceeding to read further, or you can read to the end and then come back to this point to begin all the recommended procedures. I suggest that you do it now. Take a few minutes to write on the following page your acknowledgment, your apology, and your intention to change. Then read what you have written out loud. This process will initiate within you a climate of change and a readiness to view your life here on the physical plane in a new, positive and enthusiastic way. There is so much to enjoy in life, and there are so many things to accomplish. Begin now to move away from self-punishment and into the creation of Paradise on Earth.

Resolution to Change My Philosophy

1. I acknowledge _____

_____

_____

_____

2. I apologize _____

_____

_____

_____

3. I intend _____

_____

_____

_____

Signature _____   Date _____

_____

PRACTICING APPRECIATION OF THE PHYSICAL WORLD

Once you have indicated your willingness to believe that the world and the body are good, you can develop this belief within yourself by practicing appreciation of the physical world. *Appreciation is the cornerstone of changing your attitude towards having a body and being part of the physical world.* If you practice appreciation, you will clear the way for wonderful changes in your weight and in all areas of your life.

The three main ways to practice appreciation are to: 1. regard the goodness of the physical world, 2. revise your concept of God, 3. remind yourself of your Soul's purpose.

1. REGARD THE GOODNESS OF THE PHYSICAL WORLD.

You can become more aware of the goodness of the physical world by acting on the following suggestions:

(a) *Start noticing all the good things about the world.* Really pay attention to the beauties of nature and of human achievement; really take note of the many beautiful interactions among people that take place daily. You can train your conscious and subconscious minds to view the world as good by consciously taking note of the positive things or occurrences you experience in the course of your day. These might include a beautiful sunset, an unexpected kindness performed by a co-worker, a delicious meal, a paycheck, a favorite song heard on the radio, a soothing warm shower, or any positive thing or experience that you encounter.

As you observe or experience each one, tell yourself *"This is great! It's good to be alive! Thank you, Divine Source!"* Or, *"How wonderful the world is. Thank you, Creator!"* If you adopt this simple practice, your sense of gratitude for the gift of physical existence will increase daily, and a real shift in your thinking will occur.

(b) *Become scientifically aware of the nature of the physical universe.* Read the many excellent popular works on the new physics that are available, such as those of

Michael Talbot, Gary Zukav, Fritjof Capra, and Fred Alan Wolf. You will learn how concepts from the new physics apply to our understanding of the body and how it functions. These authors and others who write on physics and consciousness show that the traditional dualistic division of matter and spirit is no longer tenable, since physical matter at its most fundamental level is nonmaterial, and matter and consciousness are part of the same vast field of energy.

Understanding the discoveries of the new physics about the nature of physical reality will inspire in you a profound appreciation of the wonders of the body and the entire physical universe. You will realize that matter is part of the spiritual continuum, and you will start to see spirit everywhere at work in what we have known as the physical plane.

(c) *Become interested in the future evolution of physical life.* As evolution has proceeded, increasingly higher levels of consciousness have been expressed in the physical world. Mineral life, plant life, animal life, and human life have all manifested and developed here. Evolution is an ongoing process, and there is every reason to believe that we are moving to even greater levels of consciousness as physical life continues to evolve. The great thinker, Jesuit priest, and paleontologist Pierre Teilhard de Chardin, who died in the 1950s, hypothesized that we are heading for a next leap in consciousness as great as the leap between ape and human consciousness. He saw the physical world as eventually evolving to an Omega Point in which all consciousnesses would be united in a new super-consciousness, which he called the Cosmic Christ.

It is impossible to think about such evolutionary potential and not feel excited about being part of the physical world. Start thinking now about the wonderful possible directions our evolution could take.

Realize that you are not part of a static or purposeless universe but of one that by its nature wants to manifest ever greater levels of perfection.

(d) *Let your immediate environment reflect the order and harmony of the physical world.* Just as we have been trashing the Earth with pollutants, and our bodies with harmful food, many of us have been trashing our homes with clutter instead of maintaining them as peaceful spaces. It is hard to regard the goodness of the physical world if your vantagepoint is blocked by mountains of clutter in your home!

Clutter is a barrier to inner peace and is thus incompatible with God-consciousness. Clutter is a frequent problem for overweight people, since as a rule we find it hard to let go. Get rid of nonessential items; clean out your closets and dispose of unused clothing and other goods. Pass along the things you aren't using to people who can use them. If you are drowning in books, magazines, catalogs, and personal papers, set up a filing system for the papers and get in the habit of disposing of the others as soon as you are done with them. Sell or give away the books that you don't expect to read or refer to again, or that you know you can always get at the public library. Make greater use of the library in general instead of buying books.

Mailing lists for catalogs have proliferated wildly; many of us receive four or five catalogs a day. This is a tremendous waste of paper and a temptation to overspend as well as a source of clutter. Decide which catalogs you really enjoy reading and phone the others to be taken off their mailing list; recycle catalogs and magazines promptly. If you have gotten out of the habit of a regular schedule for dusting and vacuuming, establish one again. Tell yourself that you are taking all these steps so that your immediate environment will reflect cosmic harmony.

Uncluttering your environment has many rewards. Orderliness on the outside promotes orderliness on the inside; your entire nervous system is soothed when your environment is gracious and uncluttered. Uncluttering also sends your subconscious mind certain vital messages, i.e., that you want order and harmony in your life, that you're the kind of person who can let go of things that no longer serve you, and that you're making room in your life for new and pleasant experiences. These messages are all significant for expediting weight loss as well as for improving your life in general. Most importantly, it will seem natural for you to view the physical world as good when your immediate space is pleasant, orderly, and harmonious.

Besides uncluttering, you can let your immediate environment reflect the harmony of the physical world by putting up pictures of beautiful natural scenery in your home and work space. You can find such pictures in calendars and magazines, or perhaps among your favorite photos. For example, I have a poster showing the hills around Assisi, Italy, in my kitchen, and another picture of the sea around the island of Rhodes in Greece above my desk. These pictures remind me of the beauty of the physical world even when I'm engaged in chores like cooking or typing.

I saw a wonderful example of this kind of reminder in an unlikely place at the city agency where I used to work. In the basement of our office building were located our copying services and our agency print shop. This basement area was windowless and smelled of acrid printing chemicals. It was also very noisy from the din of the machines and the competing blare of employees' radios.

Yet, despite the fact that it was not in any way a peaceful or gracious place, someone there had created a reminder of the goodness of physical existence. Near one of the copying machines my unknown fellow-employee had put up two pictures: one was a scene showing a cool and tranquil mountain lake, and the other was a photo of Mother Teresa smiling a radiant smile. Anyone who saw these pictures immediately felt refreshed and inspired. You can create the same kind of reminder in your unlikely places.

(e) *Reduce your focus on negative events.* Cut down on reading newspapers and watching the news: avoid TV shows and movies that capitalize on violence or on abusive humor. The media have unfortunately obscured the beauty of our physical existence by their total concentration on the criminal, horrific, or disastrous.

Tragic and ugly things do occur, but these are due to the influence of negative consciousness, both group and individual, and consciousness can be changed. Do not support the media portrayal of the world as intrinsically and unremittingly evil. Do not allow this portrayal to govern your thinking.

The above suggestions are all simple, but if you follow them it will become habitual for you to regard the physical world as good, and your appreciation and love of the physical world will flourish. Your life will also in time become easier and more pleasant, because your new, positive outlook will attract increasingly positive experiences into your life.

2. REVISE YOUR CONCEPT OF GOD.

The concept of God that we formed in childhood must change if we are to become completely free of negative thinking about the world and the body. Most of us influenced by the Judeo-Christian tradition tend to have mixed feelings about God. On the one hand, we accept intellectually that God is Spirit, All-Good and All-Powerful, the force that made us and sustains us and wants our happiness. On the other hand, we feel deep down that God is the great authoritarian avenger in the sky, eager to punish us for our transgressions. We claim that God is Spirit, but we visualize God anthropomorphically, ascribing to God all of the attributes of an earthly dictator, magnified in keeping with His omnipotent status.

Since we view the Creator as a punishing tyrant, no wonder we have the subconscious belief that we and the rest of physical creation must be evil and worthy of punishment. After all, if our own Creator doesn't love us, then who can, or should? We will never know real love and self-acceptance, nor experience a real relationship with God, for that matter, until we reject and revise any childish or limiting concepts we may have of the Divine.

Our negative view of God comes from our early religious training, given to us by teachers eager to socialize us into obedience by holding out the threat of God's retribution. If you received a strong dose of this type of religious instruction and its impact is still with you, it is important to reexamine the idea of God presented to you by these well-meaning but misguided teachers. Their idea of God came from a reading of the Bible that focused on the severe and sometimes primitive world view of its human authors, who saw divine retribution in every negative event, rather than on the divinely inspired wisdom that the Bible conveys.

As adults, we can develop an adult understanding of the Bible that moves beyond anthropomorphic projections. There are many excellent commentaries available that can help us learn from the Bible through mature understanding rather than through the distorted prism of childish fear. If your focus is on the New Testament, I would suggest you read the inspirational writings of such popular New Thought authors as Charles Fillmore, Emmet Fox, and Ernest Holmes. If the Old Testament is your focus, you can investigate the tremendously rich Jewish tradition of Kaballah, which offers an esoteric interpretation of the Hebrew scriptures.

I myself have achieved a better understanding of the Bible by contemplating Rembrandt's magnificent paintings and drawings of biblical scenes. In these works one feels directly drawn into the field of grace, love, and compassion underlying the great Bible episodes. There are many aids available for understanding scripture from mature perspectives, and we should take advantage of them if we are still locked into anthropomorphic concepts of God from childhood.

Jesus spoke of the Creator as *Abba,* an affectionate term for "Father," thus stressing God's loving and bounteous nature. Jesus was not defining God for us but was describing God's loving relationship with us in terms most meaningful to the people of that patriarchal time. No definition of God is possible; God is beyond our comprehension. With our limited minds we cannot comprehend the nature of that Unlimited Loving Source which creates, sustains, and indwells the entire cosmos yet loves each of us individually. We do know that our comprehension is inadequate and that our childish concepts must go.

Sometimes changing our language can be helpful for moving beyond childish, negative images of God. If the word God automatically evokes a punitive image for you, try using a different, less fear-provoking term when thinking or speaking about God. The word God is a cognate of the word good; you could use the terms "Supreme Good," "Loving Creator," or some similar term instead of the word God.

For many people, thinking of God as God/Goddess, or Mother/Father God has provided a broadening of outlook that has enabled them to transcend their childhood belief in a negative God. For others, a more abstract concept such as "Spirit" or "the Divine" seems to work best. The abstract term "Higher Power," so successfully used in 12-Step Programs, is one that has enabled many people to shift away from attributing negative anthropomorphic traits to God. I myself like the abstract term "Source" because it reminds me of my connection to God and the fact that God is the provider of all things.

Whichever way we do it, we must let go of our childish fears and recognize that God is loving and that God wills only good for us, including the good of a healthy, perfect-weight body. Once we truly believe in God's goodness, our appreciation of the physical world will grow in leaps and bounds, since we will realize that if the Creator of the physical world is loving and good, then the physical world, including the body, must share in this goodness and benignity.

When we truly believe that God is good, it will become easier to release the belief that the physical world is evil and the body is the prison of the soul. The physical plane is not a prison; your body is not a prison. Like all of your experiences, your body is your subconscious creation, a work of art crafted from your beliefs, emotions, and the other contents of your inner life. Changing from a childish to an adult concept of God is a major step in taking conscious charge of this otherwise subconscious process of creation.

3. REMIND YOURSELF OF YOUR SOUL'S PURPOSE.

Every morning on awakening, remind yourself of why your Higher Self or Soul Nature took physical form. Tell yourself, out loud if possible, *"I am here to creatively express Divine Perfection in the physical world. I am committed to making my body, my life and my environment a work of art. I am dedicated to the idea of Paradise on Earth."*

The cycle of overeating, excess weight, and sluggish metabolism will relax its compulsive hold on you if you take on the perspective of your Higher Self by reminding yourself of your Soul's purpose. The old subconscious view of your body as a prison will dissipate as you focus on your body's potential as a wonderful work of art. Your body will become more interesting to you; you will care more that it is properly nourished and rested.

You will also have the best of all possible motivations for losing weight. You will not be doing it to please someone else, which can work only so long as you are interested in pleasing them, nor simply to improve your health and appearance, increase ease in your life, and maximize your options, as excellent as these motivations may be. You will be losing weight as part of your great work of creating Paradise on Earth. Imbued with the perspective of your Higher Self, you will realize that Paradise begins at home, i.e. in your own body, and you will love your body in a new and altruistic way, as you would a cherished other.

As you remind yourself of your Soul's purpose, you will also begin to think about other aspects of yourself that you can enlist to express Divine Perfection in your life, such as undeveloped talents, interests that have not been followed up, or forgotten abilities. You will start to see which relationships or activities, including your job, might need changing since they do not further your Soul's purpose of creating Paradise within your life or for the world in general. You will feel less separate, more in the flow of the life force.

As you become aware of your Soul's drive to create experiences of harmony, beauty, and goodness, your life will seem magically tinged with possibility instead of just an endless round of chores. You will see the physical world as your playground rather than as a place to suffer. You will appreciate the physical world as an artist appreciates her paints, brushes, and canvases, and the artistic impulses of your Soul will find satisfaction. You will truly make peace with the physical world, and in so doing will take the first, essential step in creating a body that reflects the wholeness, grace, and perfect proportion of the Divine.

2

Understanding the

Meaning and Function

of Excess Weight

ONCE YOU MAKE PEACE with the physical world, the root cause of your weight problem will be removed. You should spend several days working intensively on this peace-making process, as described earlier in "Resolving to Change Your Philosophy" and "Practicing Appreciation of the Physical World" (pp. 23, 25). When you have made peace with the physical world, it will then become fruitful to work with changing the immediate causes, or the individual psychology, governing your particular weight situation. While the *root* cause—alienation based on the philosophy that the physical world is evil and the body is the prison of the soul— is the same for everyone, the *immediate* causes vary from individual to individual.

SUBCONSCIOUS STATEMENTS AND FUNCTIONS

These immediate causes fall into two categories: 1. *subconscious statements* of belief and self-assessment that, like the root cause, express themselves by creation of an overweight body, and 2. *subconscious functions* that are carried out by the creation of excess weight. In other words, by being overweight we are expressing something and we are accomplishing something. Our excess weight is not a random happening; it has a meaning and a function.

What are you saying by being overweight, and what does being overweight get you? It is important to decipher all of the statements you are making by being overweight, and it is also important to see how you are using excess weight to achieve a hidden, subconscious agenda. Once you fully understand what you are saying and what you are accomplishing, you will be in a position to change these underlying motivations for being overweight. You will be able to replace them with a psychology that is aligned with your Higher Self's desire to express the Divine and that is in keeping with your new commitment to creating Paradise on Earth.

REJECT GUILT

As you undertake this analysis of the immediate causes of your weight problem, it's crucial that you reject any feelings of guilt or self-recrimination you may have about being overweight. Nobody sets out to become fat; it is a subconscious process to which no guilt or blame should be attached. You must take responsibility for having created your excess weight, but taking responsibility is different from blaming yourself or feeling guilty. Guilt and blame are counterproductive; they never lead to change. Taking responsibility, on the other hand, puts you in a position to release the past, to forgive yourself and anyone else involved, and to move forward to create your perfect weight.

It's in order to take responsibility that you are going to examine your life to determine the meaning of your excess weight and the consequences your excess weight has produced for you and for the people who are close to you. Be detached and analytical in this examination, with no desire other than to uncover the truth. Take the viewpoint of a puzzle-solver, passing no judgments on yourself or anyone else. You are examining your life in order to liberate yourself, not to burden yourself further with recriminations over the past.

✍ EXCESS WEIGHT AS A PERSONAL STATEMENT

Your excess weight is not a chance occurrence. It means something; it is a form of communication in which the medium is also the message. *Being overweight is a personal statement in which you are expressing outwardly, with your body, a combination of inner beliefs and assessments regarding yourself and your life.* Some of these inner beliefs and assessments will become obvious once you begin to view your weight as a symbolic statement, while others are less readily evident. It's necessary to uncover as many as possible of these inner dicta, which make up the multiple meanings of your particular weight statement. Being overweight is a statement you are making not just to others, but also and primarily to yourself. It is a way of calling your own attention to what you need to change. The more strands of your personal statement that you unravel, the faster your progress in weight loss can be.

Pinpointing "when"

You can start your examination by pinpointing when your weight problem first developed and what the circumstances in your life were at that time. Did you become overweight after a younger sibling was born, or when you were attaining puberty, or after a disappointment or sorrow such as the loss of a job, the failure of a love relationship, or the death of a loved one? Did it start with a pregnancy weight-gain that you never recovered from, or did it come on over a long period of time as a response to daily tensions and frustrations? Did it follow a trauma such as sexual abuse? If you are someone who has apparently always been heavy, check to see whether this is really the case. Go through childhood photos to see whether you were ever at your perfect weight. If you were, you know that something must have occurred after this time that motivated you to become fat.

When you are aware of the point at which your weight problem began, the "statement" your excess weight is making often becomes obvious. You can see clearly that *your body has taken your subconscious thoughts and reactions literally and has expressed them symbolically through excess weight.* For instance, someone who gains a lot of weight after being left to raise their children alone is clearly expressing the thought "I feel burdened." Someone who becomes seriously obese after suffering physical or emotional abuse is expressing the thought "I need to have a protective barrier around me."

Even if you can't determine when your weight problem began, you can decipher the subconscious beliefs your excess weight is expressing by paying attention to the symbolism of excess weight. Our bodies are truly wonderful and deserving of praise, no matter what condition they are in! Not only do they allow us to experience the physical plane; they also make us aware of the inner dicta or authoritative statements that are governing our experience, by taking these literally and expressing them symbolically through weight.

The following is a list of the most common "statements" people make by being overweight. Many of them are interrelated, and any one instance of excess weight generally has multiple meanings. Please honestly examine your life and explore which of these statements apply to you. Remember, this is an investigative, not an accusatory process. It is also a very hopeful process, since your body will no longer have to make these statements through excess fat once you truly get the message your body has been trying to give you.

COMMON MEANINGS OF EXCESS WEIGHT

1. *I Deserve to be Punished.* As suggested in Chapter One, this belief logically follows from the philosophical concept that matter is evil and the body is a prison—a concept subconsciously held by everyone who has forgotten the true purpose of physical incarnation. Philosophical belief in one's inherent "badness" is compounded in many of us by a psychological sense of guilt arising from the circum-

stances of our lives. For example, depending on our particular situation, we may feel sexual guilt, guilt over hurting someone, guilt at surviving a loved one who has died, or other kinds of guilt and inferiority feelings that subconsciously motivate us to punish ourselves by creating a body that is a prison.

People who are severely overweight often had a strict religious upbringing or socialization that emphasized their "badness." Children often feel that they are "bad" for having committed trivial offenses, and their subconscious sense of their "badness" frequently intensifies in pre-adolescence and in teenage years as they become aware of their sexuality or experiment with sex. Girls from puritanical backgrounds sometimes develop deep shame about menstruation, and their subconscious belief that menstruation is dirty and that they should be punished for menstruating will frequently result in obesity.

Children tend to blame themselves when a death, divorce, or other upsetting reconfiguration occurs in the family. When the birth of a younger sibling naturally shifts the mother's attention away from a child, a child may believe that something wrong or unlovable about herself has caused the mother to withdraw her affection. Blaming themselves for the perceived loss of love, and feeling guilty about their hatred of the new baby, normal-weight children will often punish themselves and negatively seek attention by becoming fat.

Survivor guilt is another common trigger of obesity. The untimely death of a loved one frequently results in a sudden major weight gain by the bereaved, especially in the case of widows. Besides punishing themselves, widows in this situation are also expressing through excess weight their belief that their love life is over for good and that there is no longer any reason to try to appear attractive. Sometimes, obesity caused by survivor guilt does not appear until long after the trauma of loss. For example, adults whose parents died young will sometimes become obese after reaching the age at which their parent died, as the guilt of living longer than the parent becomes too much for them to "contain" in a normal-sized body.

The extent to which you are overweight can tell you to what extent you believe that you deserve punishment. People who are extremely fat really are imprisoned in their bodies and in many ways share the lifestyle of prisoners in jail. Like prisoners, obese people are limited in where they can go, what they can do, and whom they can associate with. Even their choice of what they can wear is limited. Like old-time prisoners, fat people are also compelled to do hard labor, carrying everywhere the heavy load of their excess weight. This self-inflicted punishment invariably becomes a vicious cycle, as self-hatred for being fat becomes another spur to punishment in addition to the guilt feelings that originally created the problem.

2. *I'm a Prisoner of Circumstances.* This belief is often at work among people whose lives have been altered by tragedy or a reversal of fortune, or people who have habitually experienced a lack of financial resources. As discussed in Chapter One, the body can express belief in your prisoner-hood by becoming a prison of fat.

3. *I Feel Confined.* If you habitually feel this way, your subconscious will accept this feeling as a command and will confine you in the most direct way it knows, by creating a heavy and confining body.

4. *I Feel Burdened.* This is a common self-assessment found among people who are tied to jobs, family, or other responsibilities that make heavy demands on them. The body tends to take this feeling literally and manifests a burden of excess weight. This is especially common among nurses, social workers, clergy, or others in the helping professions.

5. *I Feel Weighed Down* (by woes or responsibilities). Similar to "I feel burdened."

6. *I've Taken on More than My Share.* Also similar, but with the added dimension of believing that your lot in life is particularly heavy in comparison with other people's. Your body "adds dimension" accordingly by becoming significantly heavier than other bodies.

7. *I Deserve Compensation* (for a great loss). Many people feel this way after losing a love, a job, a home, etc. If you hold on to this desire for compensation, your subconscious, with its nonrational but inexorable logic, can conclude that you want a great gain and thus impel you to become fat. Interestingly, the root of the word "compensation" is the Latin verb *pendere,* to weigh.

8. *I Feel Deprived of Love.* Similar to "I deserve compensation." *Feeling deprived of love is a statement/motivation underlying all cases of obesity,* especially obesity originating in childhood. Love is the nourishment of the psyche, as food is the nourishment of the body. When the psyche feels deprived of love, the body calls attention to this sense of deprivation by wildly overeating.

9. *I Don't Want to Lose Any More.* Also similar to "I deserve compensation," this subconscious statement can lead to particularly stubborn weight problems following the loss of love, security, or other sources of happiness. Your body expresses your inner desire not to lose any more by gaining weight and tenaciously holding on to it.

10. *I'm Fed Up.* If you feel fed up with your life in general or with a particular situation, your subconscious mind will impel you to express this by stuffing yourself to the maximum.

11. *I Feel Stuck.* People often feel this way when they are in a situation that they know should be changed yet they cannot see their way to making changes. If this feeling is a habitual one, the body will express it by making stuck the bioenergy that would otherwise be circulating freely and

evenly throughout the body. Excess weight develops where the energy is stuck.

12. *I'm Not Free to Move On.* Similar to "I feel stuck." The subconscious feeling of not being free to move on frequently arises where there is a sense of incompletion regarding a past relationship. Important conversations that were never held, emotions that were never expressed, or a general lack of closure in a past relationship can all make you feel that you are not free to continue on with your life. Your body will respond to this feeling by not allowing your bioenergy to circulate freely.

13. *My Life Isn't Going Anywhere.* Also similar to "I feel stuck." This belief, which is associated with feelings of boredom and a lack of expectations, is generally the cause of that extra 20 pounds that refuses to budge despite all your efforts at dieting.

14. *I Feel Immobilized.* This feeling represents an extreme case of feeling stuck and leads to serious obesity problems. It often occurs after someone has been overwhelmed by a disastrous event in his or her life.

15. *I Shall Not Be Moved.* Clinging to anger or resentment, rigid insistence on one's opinions, holding on to the past, or other forms of mental and emotional intransigence can result in extreme heaviness and, if unchecked, to the eventual inability to move about freely.

16. *I Won't Let Go.* If you won't let go or drop your old resentments, anger, bitterness, guilt, and other negative emotions, your body won't let go of excess weight. Your body is the faithful reflection of your psyche and can only act in keeping with your inner attitudes.

17. *I'm Full of Pent-up Emotions.* Emotions are energy. If your emotions are constantly pent-up rather than appropriately released, your life force or bioenergy will not be able to circulate properly. The result will be the produc-

tion of fat, which may be defined as excess stored or pent-up energy.

18. *I'm Out of Circulation Now.* This self-assessment may be at work if you have gained a lot of weight since marrying. You may feel that you're out of circulation if you believe that your marriage is restricting you rather than increasing your enjoyment of life. People also can feel that they're out of circulation because their lives have gotten into a rut. Always responsive to your thoughts and eager to express them, your body may slow down the circulation of your bioenergy accordingly, thus producing fat.

19. *My Love Life Is Over Now.* A variant of "I'm out of circulation." This belief is held by many people who perceive themselves as being too bereaved, too disillusioned, too old, or too unlovable to find a new partner. The body reduces life force, or bioenergy circulation, accordingly. It also obediently overeats in order to minimize the possibility of a new relationship by creating a barrier.

20. *I Am Unlovable.* If you feel unlovable, your body can respond by taking on a shape that is unlovable by the standards of our society, whatever we may think of these standards. Feeling unlovable creates a vicious cycle, since it produces a barrier of fat that makes it harder for you to find love, and your original feeling of unlovableness is confirmed and intensified.

21. *I Demand to Be Noticed.* The body can respond to an insistent desire for attention by gaining weight, since weight is something highly visible and people always notice when one is overweight. Of course the subconscious mind, and thus the body, cannot distinguish between positive and negative attention. *The desire for attention underlies all problems of excess weight;* in addition to whatever else it might be stating, excess weight is always a plea for attention. The more the weight, the greater the plea.

22. *I Want to Throw My Weight Around.* Like the simpler demand to be noticed, an aggressive desire to have power over others or to dominate them can frequently result in obesity. The body will symbolically express your desire to throw your weight around by producing lots and lots of excess weight. Two very extreme examples of this are represented by the stereotypes of the fat, ruthless capitalist and the fat, violent gangster. Many of us who are not ruthless or violent, however, unfortunately also express our desire to throw our weight around by becoming fat when we fail to find proper channels for our aggressiveness.

23. *I'm No Lightweight.* People who feel that they are not taken seriously will often be subconsciously motivated to gain weight as an expression of their importance. Fear of thinness (which will be discussed in more detail in a later chapter) often comes from the subconscious fear of being regarded as a "lightweight," a person of no consequence.

24. *I'm into Self-Aggrandizement.* A subconscious desire for self-aggrandizement can arise from feelings of inferiority and insecurity and can have harmful weight repercussions. Latin is once again a key, since *aggrandize* comes from the Latin *aggrandare,* "to make bigger." If you want to become bigger than others in importance, you may express this symbolically by becoming bigger in weight than others as well.

25. *I'm Too Big for the Small Role in Life I've Been Given.* People who have no outlet in their environment for their talents or aspirations often feel this way. If they don't take active steps to broaden their horizons, their bodies may express their sense of being caught in a narrow milieu by broadening in size.

26. *I Want More Space.* Similar to "I'm too big for my small role." If you feel that you don't have enough scope for your talents, enough room to maneuver, or even enough

living space, your body may express your desire for more space by taking up more space physically.

27. *I've Been Waiting and Waiting.* Your subconscious mind can't distinguish between "wait" and "weight." If instead of creating interesting experiences in your life you are always waiting for something to happen, your subconscious mind will impel you to express this excessive waiting by gaining excess weight. This is especially true if deep down you are waiting for the perfect mate to find you, and you feel that the wait is interminable.

28. *I Feel Separate from Everybody Else.* A sense of separateness can arise from fear of other people, fear of intimacy, feelings of unworthiness, or the belief that one has been singled out for unhappiness or deprivation. People who feel separate from others or different from everybody else will often express this physically by separating themselves from others by a barrier of fat.

29. *I Don't Fit In.* Obesity frequently results from the belief that one is so intrinsically different from others that one doesn't "fit in." The significant number of psychics who are obese is attributable to this belief. People who have felt outside the mainstream since childhood can express their sense of not "fitting in" by becoming too fat to fit into normal-sized clothing and, in extreme cases, normal-sized furniture or cars.

30. *There's a Barrier to My Happiness.* If you subconsciously focus on barriers to your happiness (such as lack of funds, your age, or some detail of your appearance), your body will express your barrier consciousness by creating a barrier of fat.

31. *I Need Protection.* Excess weight is a protective barrier that you put up between yourself and other people or between yourself and life in general because you feel threatened in some way. Job anxiety, financial stress,

feelings of being sexually threatened, or other sources of insecurity can all result in a deeply felt need for protection. This need also commonly arises when people feel that their mates are losing interest in them or that some other possible loss of love may be at hand. The need for protection lies behind the frequent occurrence of weight gain after a major life trauma. People whose thinking is very dualistically oriented may moreover subconsciously conclude that if a traumatic event occurred when they were thin, then protection will be insured if they remain fat. Unless this conclusion is corrected, their subconscious will vigorously resist any attempt to lose weight.

32. *I Have No Control over What Happens in My life.* People frequently feel this way after tragedy, disaster or emotional devastation has struck in their lives. This sense of having no control may be expressed by losing control over one's food intake and wildly overeating. By thus letting your weight get out of control, you are making the statement that you have been unable to control the course of your life as you would have wished.

33. *I Have a Hunger That Can't Be Filled.* When people have experienced a terrible loss or are undergoing intense emotional or creative frustration, they will often subconsciously feel that they have a hunger that can't be filled. The body takes them literally, and they overeat constantly yet are constantly hungry.

34. *I'm Dissatisfied with My Life.* A lesser version of "I have a hunger that can't be filled." Dissatisfaction often expresses itself through endless nibbling.

35. *I Have Something to Hide.* This belief is often found among preteens who are embarrassed by their developing bodies, adolescents who are embarrassed about sexual matters, and people who feel guilty about transgressions of the past, whether these were serious or only appeared serious to them at the time. In the logic of the subcon-

scious, a covering of excess weight is a natural response to and expression of the sense of having something to hide.

36. *I Have to Hide Who I Am in Order to Be Safe.* This subconscious belief, which generally results in many protective layers of fat, is common among people who have been sexually abused or harassed, or among others who for various reasons fear sex or fear being perceived as a sexually attractive being. This belief can stem from nonsexual fears as well. You may have deep-rooted fears about revealing your true nature if you grew up in an environment where you would have been harassed for appearing to be as spiritual, intellectual, powerful, or accomplished as you really were. Past life experiences of harassment can also contribute to a subconscious desire to hide oneself in the safe and sure disguise of fat.

37. *Things Have Gone beyond the Limit.* People who feel that they have been pushed beyond the limits of their endurance, whether through excess work, worries, misfortunes, or the demands of other people, often express this feeling by eating beyond the natural limit of their appetite. They thus create a body size that is far beyond the limits of normalcy.

38. *I Wish I Were a Baby Again.* Fat is often subconsciously equated with baby fat and thus with the baby state, or state of non-responsibility. A child who becomes fat after the birth of a sibling is subconsciously endeavoring to compete with the new baby by becoming baby-like again. Boys and girls who become fat as teenagers are often expressing the desire to return to the perceived safety and innocence of babyhood. When we are fat as adults, no matter what else we are expressing, we are stating our subconscious nostalgia for a time when no demands were made on us and all our needs were met.

39. *I'm as Harmless as a Baby.* This is a statement made primarily, though not exclusively, by men who are obese.

People whose fat looks very soft and babyish (as opposed to the tougher, more solid "gangster" type of fat) are making the statement that they are no threat to anyone. Such obesity may occur as a survival stratagem adopted in childhood in response to a particular perceived danger, or it may result from the beliefs that the world in general is a combative, threatening place and that one's best chance for survival lies in appearing totally harmless. It can also arise from the subconscious belief that one must maintain a babylike, non-threatening appearance because one's aggressiveness would wreak havoc if it were ever allowed to come to the surface.

40. *I'm Showing Solidarity with Someone Else Who Is Fat.* If you have a problem with excess weight, and your mother, father, aunt, etc., also had one, you have experienced a strong identification with that particular family member and are literally showing "solidarity" with them by being fat. This can happen even if you feel angry with that particular relative or are completely alienated from them on the conscious level. Aversion is as strong a bond as attraction, and both can result in intense identifications that can lead to serious weight problems. The fat in such cases may be especially solid and hard to lose.

41. *I've Lost My Sense of Proportion.* By manifesting a weight that is disproportionate for your height and bone structure, you've alerted yourself to the fact that you have overemphasized or neglected certain aspects of your life, whether these be your job, a love affair, family responsibilities, etc. Disproportionate attention or inattention to any aspect of your life can result in disproportionate size, since it is the natural tendency of the body to reflect your mental outlook. In addition, excess weight is symbolic of the tendency to overreact emotionally and blow things out of proportion. Exaggerated emotions tend to create exaggerated weight. One reason people often lose weight after they start to meditate is that meditation lessens the

tendency to emotionally over react. When a sense of proportion is regained emotionally, the body follows suit by returning to its proper proportions.

42. *I Refuse to Conform to Your Expectations.* Being overweight is generally a statement of subconscious rebellion. In some instances, overweight people are rebelling against society's conventions, including the convention that women must conform to certain standards of thinness if they are to be considered beautiful. In other cases, people are expressing their rebelliousness against their family members' expectations of them, whatever these expectations may be. The thought "I refuse to conform" can make one's form, or size, the outer locus and expression of an inner attitude of rebelliousness. Intense feelings of rebelliousness can produce extreme obesity.

43. *I Want to Be Loved for Who I Am, Not What I Look Like.* This subconscious desire is held by many people who are highly romantic or idealistic in nature. At first glance this desire seems to be a spiritually elevated one, based on an awareness of the possibility of unconditional love. On further examination, though, one can see that it is another harmful instance of dualistic thinking, in which the soul and body are viewed as being in opposition to each other. As Chapter One stresses, this type of thinking leads to the subconscious conclusion that the body is the prison of the soul, and the body responds by making of itself a prison of excess weight.

44. *My Life Is a Drag or My life Is a Downer.* Any such beliefs about the heaviness of life can impel you to gain excess weight. Heavy thoughts produce heavy bodies; light thoughts produce bodies of perfect weight and proportion. If your view of your life is pessimistic rather than upbeat, your body will comply with your view by dragging you down with excess weight.

TAKING STOCK OF YOUR STATEMENTS

To understand what your excess weight means—that is, what you are expressing by being overweight—go through the above statements and take note of all the ones that apply to you. Many of the statements are interrelated, and it's easy to see how one would flow from the other, such as "I feel burdened" and "I feel stuck." Some seem to contradict each other, such as "I demand to be noticed" and "I have something to hide." Pay attention to all the statements that ring a bell with you, even if they seem contradictory. Your excess weight has multiple meanings, since the human psyche is so complex, and this multiplicity can include even the most contradictory and seemingly unrelated subconscious thoughts and feelings.

ANY OTHERS?

Also see whether any statements occur to you that have not been given above. Additional statements may tend to come to mind once you start thinking about your weight and your body as a symbolic outer expression of inner dicta. If feelings of guilt or shame should surface during this process, thank them for coming to the surface but firmly instruct them to leave. Tell them *"I have serious work to do, and I cannot be sidetracked by unproductive feelings now."*

When you have gone through this process, you will be aware of the inner beliefs and attitudes that you have been expressing by being fat. Other people who held these attitudes might have expressed them differently; for example, someone else who felt burdened might have expressed this by developing round shoulders or back problems rather than by becoming fat. You have expressed your negative thoughts by becoming overweight because your deeply held philosophical belief that the body is the prison of the soul has made weight your focus of expression.

Now that your negative inner dicta have come to your conscious notice, you can give them all the attention they require. You can observe them, think about them, and then decide to change them or change to a harmless way of expressing them. In either case, you have to change.

◯ MAKING NEW STATEMENTS: AFFIRMATIONS

Begin by selecting some statements to work on and figuring out where you can make appropriate changes in the outer circumstances of your life so that these statements will no longer apply as much. For example, if you have been feeling burdened, think of ways in which you can ease your situation. Adopt the attitude that there is always something you can do to make your life easier.

Ask for help from friends, relatives, or social service agencies. Lighten your schedule as much as possible, cutting back on burdensome extraneous activities or even on overscheduled pleasurable activities that are increasing pressure on you by taking up too much time. Provide yourself with a relaxation period every day.

Learn to meditate, since meditation enhances purposefulness and puts you on automatic pilot for maximum efficiency and maximum organization. The number of hours available to you every day will expand if you begin the day with meditation. Get up earlier in the morning if you have to in order to meditate; in just a short time you will look forward to this early rising because you will associate it with the pleasure of meditation.

DO THE NEW

If you are feeling stuck, get things moving in your life again. Alter your daily routine in some way, and remind yourself that you're doing this as a sign that your life is starting to change. Even a small shift in your outer routine can precipitate an important inner shift in consciousness. You can take brisk walks, take up a new pursuit, or take a vacation to a new place. Learning something new is an especially powerful message to your subconscious that you want your life to start moving again. Planning a trip to someplace new can bring a whole new influx of energy into your life.

If you feel that you are out of circulation, remind yourself that you are part of a larger whole and that you have a role to play within this whole, promoting the free flow of connectedness and universal well-being. Start acting like someone who is in circulation; get a new haircut, buy something new to wear, attend group events and volunteer for group projects. Start the day with the attitude that you are in the flow of life and that something wonderful is about to happen.

There is always something in your situation that you can change for the better by behaving differently. And, by changing your external patterns of behavior, you can bring about the crucial change in your inner dicta that must be made if you wish to attain your perfect weight. You can also change your inner dicta by consciously substituting new statements for old ones. External and internal phenomena are part of the same cycle, so it doesn't matter if you approach your change from the external or the internal level, as long as the internal level is affected.

KEEP IT SPIRITUAL

New, positive statements that one consciously adopts in place of the old, harmful inner dicta are known as affirmations. Affirmations work best when they focus on yourself as a spiritual being, since as a spiritual being you have the potential to create whatever good thing you wish to have in your life, whether this be good health, financial success, a wonderful love relationship, or your perfect weight.

If you've had a severe weight problem, it may be hard for you to believe that the everyday you, you the personality, can lose excess weight; but who can doubt the power of you the Higher Self?! Nothing is impossible to the Soul or Higher Self, which is the aspect of you most illuminated by spiritual awareness and most linked to the Divine. The more you can remind yourself of your spiritual aspect and your natural right to Divine help, the more successful your affirmations will be.

You can replace your old statements with affirmations based on spiritual power. Daily use of such affirmations will change your psyche so that your body will no longer be under a subconscious requirement to manifest excess weight. The following suggested affirmations will help you create a new and beneficent inner environment. Before each affirmation I've indicated in parentheses the old statements that it can replace:

(*I Deserve to Be Punished.*) I reject self-punishment completely. I fulfill my Divine destiny to thrive and be happy. I accept God's forgiveness, and I forgive myself and others with full grace and mercy. I can do this because I am a spiritual being. My body is a Divine creation, so I value my body and allow it to be completely well and free. My body is always good and worthy of praise.

(*I'm a Prisoner of Circumstances. I Feel Confined.*) I enjoy the freedom of a child of God. There is always a way out that is to the benefit of all concerned. I accept the perfect solution now.

(*I Feel Burdened. I Feel Weighed Down.*) I release all burdens to the Higher Power. Because I have cast my burdens on the Higher Power, nothing can weigh me down. I am light and free, through the power of the Divine.

(I've Taken on More than My Share.) Because I am a spiritual being help is always available to me. I do what I can, and my Source provides help for the rest. Now that I accept Divine help, my life is becoming easier and more joyful. I give thanks for the Divine gift of my new-found freedom.

(I Deserve Compensation. I Don't Want to Lose Any More. I Feel Deprived.) I bless and release the past. I am a spiritual being, and all the love, nurture, and security I need is always available to me. I allow my Source to bring everything I need into my life now, in ways that are perfect for me. Wonderful things are happening now.

(I'm Fed Up.) As a spiritual being, change is always possible for me. I now allow my life to change to one that is easier and more rewarding. With Divine help, I return to the center of calm within, and I look forward to wonderful new life circumstances. I am open to new ideas and opportunities.

(I Feel Stuck. I'm Not Free to Move On. My Life Isn't Going Anywhere. I Feel Immobilized. I'm Out of Circulation.) As a spiritual being, I am part of the mainstream of life. I open myself fully to the Divine flow of freedom and self-expression. I let the Higher Power circulate in my life now to create perfect circumstances. Through Divine Grace my life is improving now in every way.

(I Shall Not Be Moved. I Won't Let Go.) It's time to give up the past and look forward to the future. I can do it because I am a spiritual being with endless access to Divine help. I now bless and release the past. I safely release all of my old, negative emo-

tions. I am open to peaceful new thought patterns and wonderful new experiences. I am flexible in my thinking and supple in my body. Thank you, great Source, for putting me on a new path of peace, health, and beauty.

(I'm Full of Pent-up Emotions.) As a spiritual being, I am endlessly creative and inventive. I thus find ways to release my negative emotions fully and safely. I am cleansed and balanced now. New ways for positive self-expression come into my life, as I choose to serve the Divine Artist within.

(My Love Life Is Over Now. I Am Unlovable.) As a spiritual being, my nature is love. By focusing on my true nature, I am attracting abundant love into my life. There is no limit to love in the universe; plenty of love is available to me now, and I call it into my life. Through the power of Divine Love, wonderful love is coming to me now.

(I Demand to Be Noticed. I Want to Throw My Weight Around.) I can let go of the desire to control and still get what I need. I am a spiritual being, so I am worthy of attention, power, and respect. I now allow myself to experience these in wonderful ways, and as a normal-weight person. Through the power of the Divine within, my needs are met easily and harmlessly, with full respect for others. I am a gracious star in the movie of my life!

(I'm No Lightweight.) Because I am a spiritual being, I can be a normal weight and still be taken seriously. I can be a normal weight and still be powerful. By calling on Divine Power, I now find ways of expressing my intelligence and authority which are benign to all, including myself and my

body. I recognize my worth, and I increasingly receive respect and recognition from others. Thank you, Great Creator, for bringing me the perfect showcase for my talents now.

(I'm into Self-Aggrandizement. I'm Too Big for the Small Role I've Been Given in Life. I Want More Space.) I give up the need to dominate, and I allow Divine Power to have full sway. By cooperating with Divine Power, I now have all the space and scope I need to express myself perfectly. I receive recognition and appreciation from others in ways that are beneficial to all. Wonderful opportunities are mine now.

(I've Been Waiting and Waiting.) I stop waiting and start creating. I ask God's help in creating my body and my life to be lively, free and joyful. Great things are happening now. I *can* lose weight!

(I Feel Separate from Everybody Else. I Don't Fit In.) As a child of God, I acknowledge my connection to everybody and everything. I am now willing to join the mainstream of life. With the help of Divine Grace, I allow myself to experience happiness, fulfillment, and a sense of belonging. Wherever I am is the right place for me to be. I'm part of the mainstream now, and it's wonderful.

There's a Barrier to My Happiness.) I am a child of God and thus good enough to deserve happiness. I cooperate as Divine Grace dissolves any barriers to my happiness now. I realize that my happiness does not depend on any particular person or event; it can come about in a multitude of different ways, in accordance with the grace and creativity of Divine Providence. I am open to receiving happiness now, and I look forward to the future. May all beings be happy, including me!

(I Need Protection.) I get over the experiences of the past; past experiences no longer keep me down. Recognizing my Divine origin, I begin my life anew in complete confidence and safety. Through the power of the Divine, I am always safe. It is safe for me to reveal myself. It is safe for me to love. It is safe for me to be a normal weight. I can have a safe and happy sexual relationship. Divine Protection flows through me and around me at all times, so that I everywhere encounter safety and acceptance. My self-confidence and sense of security increase every day, thanks to my new awareness of God's omnipresent love. Divine love is my shield and companion.

(I Have No Control over What Happens in My Life. Things Have Gone Beyond the Limit.) I invoke God's help to restore order and balance in my life. I open myself to allow Divine Order to transform my life, weight, and experiences now. Things are quickly and easily changing for the better. Order, harmony, and balance prevail, through the power of the Most High. I give thanks that my life is improving now.

(I Have a Hunger That Can't Be Filled. I'm Dissatisfied.) Divine Mind knows exactly what I need to be satisfied, and Divine Power can provide it in a perfect form. I now prepare myself for true satisfaction. The Divine Provider is bringing me all the love and appreciation I desire. The perfect avenue of self-expression is opening to me now. I am contented and at peace.

(I Have Something to Hide.) I have nothing to hide, since in Divine Mind I am always innocent. Errors of the past are washed away in the waters of forgiveness. I accept and give thanks for my new

beginning. I let the beauty of my body be revealed now, knowing that I am always surrounded by the safety and protection of the Divine. Through Divine Protection, it is safe for me to be my perfect weight. It is safe for me to be attractive. I am always innocent and safe.

(*I Have to Hide Who I Am in Order to Be Safe.*) The truth is that I'm a beautiful, powerful spiritual being. This is my only true identity, and it is always safe for me to express it. I no longer fear or hide my power and my beauty; I let my true Self be revealed. I let my body be perfect-weight and attractive. I can handle other people's recognition of how beautiful and powerful I am. I accept my body as a superb medium for the expression of my Divine qualities. I am always safe, through the power of the Most High.

(*I Wish I Were a Baby Again.*) I place myself under Divine protection, so it is safe for me to accept adulthood. I am happy to be an adult now. I rely on the power of God, and so my needs are met easily and with full abundance. I enjoy the freedom, the pleasures, the responsibilities, and the opportunities of being an adult. I accept them all as a Divine gift. With God's help I have a mature and confident attitude toward life.

(*I'm as Harmless as a Baby.*) As a spiritual being, I am strong, powerful, confident and mature. I allow these qualities of my Soul to manifest in my life now, through the power of the Almighty. Through Divine Power, it is safe for me to show my strength. It is safe for me to be an adult. With God's help I use my power wisely and well.

(I'm Showing Solidarity with Someone Else Who Is Fat.) Through the power of the Most High, I realize that I am my own person now. I am not my ———— (whichever relative you have been showing solidarity with). I bless my ————, and I pray that any negative connections between us will be cleared up now. I identify with the health, beauty, and balance of my Higher Self. I accept my Divine destiny to thrive and be happy.

(I've Lost My Sense of Proportion.) I'm regaining my sense of proportion now. I can do it, because with God all things are possible. My lifestyle is becoming balanced and harmonious. I pay the right amount of time and attention to all my needs and all the facets of my life. My emotions also are balanced; through the power of the Divine I always react appropriately and with a sense of proportion. I give thanks that Divine Order prevails in my inner and outer worlds. It is wonderful to be back in balance now!

(I Refuse to Conform to Your Expectations.) Through the power of the Divine, I express my individuality in ways that are beneficial to all, including my body. I choose peaceful means to display my uniqueness and share my opinions. I respect others and I receive respect. Divine Guidance leads me to the perfect outlet for my originality and independence. Thank you, Great Creator, for the great new path that opens to me now.

(I Want to Be Loved for Who I Am, Not What I Look Like.) I acknowledge that body and soul are one continuum of Divine Light. My body is good and is always worthy of praise. I am at peace with my body. I allow it to be as healthy and attractive as

possible, as a reflection of the order and beauty of the Divine. Through the power of the Divine, it is safe for me to be attractive. Through the power of the Divine, I can have an attractive body and attract a mate who understands and cherishes my soul. I give up dualistic thinking now. I am committed to a mature understanding of the integration of body and soul.

(My Life Is a Drag. My Life Is a Downer.) I am changing my attitude towards life now. I accept my life as a Divine gift to be enjoyed and appreciated. I am committed to having a long, healthy, happy life. I rely on the Divine within to fill my life with experiences of love, fun, prosperity, and creative self-expression. I give thanks now for the remarkable gift of life!

Select the affirmation that you think would be most helpful for you at this time and work with it intensively for a two-week period. Every day, read the entire affirmation out loud at least five times, accepting every sentence of it with heartfelt conviction. When reciting your affirmation, always have at the back of your mind the awareness that the universe is fluid, that we are evolving towards perfection, and that everything therefore can easily change for the better.

The physical universe really is always in flux; even the natural objects that seem so solid to us, such as a chair or a table, are actually full of molecules in motion. Our bodies too are always changing; after every seven years, every cell in our body has been replaced with a new one. We can take advantage of the tendency to change that is inherent in our universe to change our inner state. Changing our negative inner world to a higher, more evolutionary one may be seen as part of the natural order of things and does not have to be difficult. Affirmations can propel us into the river of personal change and direct our course in the way we would like it to go.

Sometimes negative feelings and objections to an affirmation can arise in us when we are using it. For example, we might affirm *"I am contented and at peace"* and suddenly realize how very anxious or unhappy we are. We might think of all the reasons that we can't possibly feel contented or at peace. When such thoughts or feelings arise, simply observe them, and be glad that they have come to the surface. Realize that the affirmation is flushing out your old inner dicta.

AFFIRMATIONS GO HIGHER

Even if the words of your affirmation do not seem like an accurate description of your current state, know that they are true on the spiritual level and that your physical reality will soon reflect this newly apprehended spiritual truth. For example, you can accept the phrase "I am contented and at peace" as true, even if right now you feel dissatisfied, because being contented and at peace is always true of you at the Soul level.

If you fill your consciousness with this higher truth rather than with your old statements, your current state will shift to reflect your higher consciousness, and you will become contented and at peace. Your affirmation is a description of a higher level of being, an invocation of this higher truth into your current experience, and an instruction to your subconscious mind to manifest that which has been invoked.

If there is one particular sentence in the affirmation that especially appeals to you, repeat it to yourself silently or out loud a number of times throughout the day. You can also write out the affirmation in its entirety, if this appeals to you. Make a real commitment to working seriously with the affirmation for the two-week period; it requires commitment, diligence, and pleasurable effort for the new flow of consciousness to do its wonderful work.

REEVALUATE THE AFFIRMATION

At the end of the two weeks, take a couple of days off from using the affirmation and decide whether to continue with it for another two-week period or to select another affirmation. Base your decision to continue on whether you are enjoying the affirmation and whether you feel enthusiastic about its potential to help you change. You need to have a sense of enjoyment and a sense of expectancy in order for the affirmation to be effective. If your affirmation still seems like fun and feels transformative, continue with it until you feel that a shift has been accomplished. Select another one if you feel that a shift has already occurred, if your enjoyment is waning, or simply if you are strongly drawn to another one. Reevaluate every two weeks. Rely on your Higher Self to help you select the affirmation that is the best for you at this time.

Don't worry about having to use all of the affirmations that correspond to your old inner dicta. You might eventually use them, or you might not. You will find that by replacing even a few of your old statements with affirmations, the other negative inner statements will automatically change. Continue using these affirmations for two-week periods until that marvelous time when your body will express through perfect weight your psyche's new sense of self-worth and well-being.

THE FUNCTION OF EXCESS WEIGHT

Just as you must determine what you have been saying by being overweight, you must also determine what you have been accomplishing. What is the function of your excess weight in your life? What has it gotten you?

As we have seen, being overweight expresses our inner dicta and also fulfills them. To this extent the meaning and function of our excess weight are one and the same. We believe that we need to punish ourselves, attract attention, create protection, hide our true selves, etc., and our being fat both states these needs and achieves them as goals.

Our excess weight also serves another function, however. This is as a tool of control in the dynamics of our relationships with other people. We frequently use excess weight to fulfill a hidden agenda of annoying, frustrating, or otherwise controlling those who are close to us. We cannot be free from excess weight until we relinquish its use as a tool to manipulate other people or to score against them.

REVIEW YOUR RELATIONSHIPS

You must review your relationships with family members and friends to determine whether you are using your excess weight for purposes of manipulation, revenge, or other attempts at control. Once again, adopt an attitude of objectivity and nonjudgment before beginning your review. To set you thinking about the way excess weight can function in relationship dynamics, here are some examples from experiences of people I have known (names have been changed to preserve confidentiality, and some cases are composites):

> 1. KATHLEEN is married to Jim, a man from a large, close-knit family of brothers and sisters who enjoy getting together most weekends during the summer at their parents' lakeside cabin. Kathleen loathes Jim's brothers and sisters; they drink too heavily, and they make her feel like an outsider since they are an extremely athletic family and she is not very good at sports. Jim, on the other hand, feels very close to his siblings and thoroughly enjoys being with them. Like them, he loves swimming and boating at the lake.
> Kathleen feels that Jim is more loyal to his original family than to her and bitterly resents this. She

does not want to risk alienating her husband by refusing to go to the lake; besides, she broods, if he were really sensitive to her needs, he would understand her feelings without her having to make a big issue about his family. Over time, Kathleen gains so much weight that she no longer feels comfortable appearing in a bathing suit. "Look," she tells Jim, "there's no way I can go to the lake looking like this." Kathleen is so upset about her weight and makes such a fuss about it that she and Jim stop going to the cabin.

Kathleen's excess weight has enabled her to separate herself and Jim from his family, but it has been at the cost of unhappiness on her part, and feelings of conflict and resentment in Jim.

2. MELANIE has discovered that her husband Gary has been unfaithful to her. Gary has ended his relationship with the other woman, but Melanie cannot get over it. She is still in love with Gary, and at the same time she is furiously angry with him. She doesn't want a divorce, yet she feels that Gary's infidelity has created an insuperable barrier to any kind of emotional unity between them again. Melanie longs for the old days when their relationship was at its romantic peak, but the thought of having sex with Gary now turns her off completely.

Melanie starts eating heavily, and in a short time gains a substantial amount of weight. Gary begins to lose interest in having sex with her. Through her excess weight, Melanie has succeeded in distancing Gary, but she feels terrible about her weight and she is angrier with Gary than ever. She feels thoroughly rejected now as well as betrayed.

3. MIKE works in the stockroom of a store that is part of a major electronics chain. He was extremely

heavy but has recently lost a lot of weight. The store manager tells Mike that he is considering him for a promotion to a sales position that will open up in a few months when one of the sales staff retires. Mike has always wanted to work in sales, and he is excited at the prospect. At the same time he lacks self-confidence and worries that he will not be able to make the grade as a salesman. He begins overeating again and is obese by the time the position opens.

The manager, who now thinks that Mike's appearance would have a negative impact on his ability to generate sales, passes over Mike and gives the position to someone else instead. Mike feels furious and bitter. He also has a conflicting feeling of relief. Part of him believes that he would have made a good salesman, but part of him thinks it's just as well that he didn't get the job, since now he won't have to compete. At quite a cost to himself, Mike has used excess weight to manipulate his manager into selecting someone else, thus extricating himself from a potentially threatening position.

4. TERRY is a teenager whose parents are divorced. Because her mother is ill, she is temporarily living with her father, her stepmother, and her stepbrother, who is quite a bit younger than Terry. Terry is unhappy there and resents the fact that her father seems to care more about his stepson than about her. She has always had a weight problem, but in these circumstances her eating goes completely out of control.

Terry's father is upset about her obesity, and it becomes the subject of heated arguments between the two of them. The house is in a constant state of uproar, with lots of shouting, slamming of doors, and, on Terry's part, tears of recrimination.

After every scene, Terry feels bitterly unhappy and unloved, yet strangely relieved and exhilarated.

Through her obesity she has found a way to deeply upset her father and thus to some extent equalize the balance of power between them.

5. NICOLE and her sister Janet have a long-standing rivalry. Janet is married to an extremely wealthy physician and has two beautiful children. She does not work outside the home, but nevertheless has a housekeeper and a full-time babysitter. Nicole is not married and is afraid that she will never have children. "Janet has everything, and I have nothing," she often thinks bitterly. Nicole has an unpleasant commute to a job she dislikes, and on dark, cold winter mornings often thinks about how unfair it is that she has to get up and go to work while Janet is no doubt still asleep in her comfortable home.

As Nicole continues to be dissatisfied with her life, she begins to overeat more and more. In time she develops an extreme case of obesity. She becomes so heavy that she can no longer fit into her car. Nicole has to give up her job. She feels mortified, angry, and thoroughly sorry for herself, but at the same time she feels a sense of satisfaction in knowing that, like Janet, she no longer has to get up and go to work.

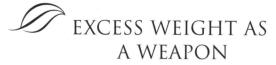

EXCESS WEIGHT AS A WEAPON

None of the people in the examples given above consciously set out to become fat in order to thwart, manipulate, anger, or score against someone else. Nevertheless, becoming fat was their subconsciously chosen way to achieve these ends. They wielded their excess weight as a powerful weapon in an overt or undeclared war of wills.

Becoming fat served the dual function of *a)* expressing and fulfilling their need for self-punishment and their sense of being stuck, and *b)* controlling others.

RELATIONSHIP QUESTIONS

Having read through these examples, it's now time for you to examine your own relationships to see how your excess weight has affected their dynamics. To do this, consider your most important relationships and ask yourself the following questions:

1. Does my being overweight allow me to get out of doing something that I don't want to do?

2. Does my being overweight enable me to have things go the way I want?

3. Does my being overweight upset or annoy someone?

4. Does my being overweight allow me to even the score with someone?

If you answer yes to any of these questions, realize that you have been using your excess weight as a weapon in your relationships with others. Resolve to stop this and to set about finding ways of dealing with other people that cause harm to no one, yourself included.

In the examples given above, for instance, Kathleen could have been honest with Jim and tried to work out some kind of compromise. Mike could have used the months before the new position opened to work on developing self-confidence; as a starting point, he could have asked the manager why he thought he would make a successful salesman and then worked on cultivating those qualities. Melanie could have sought counseling to resolve her very deeply divided feelings about her husband. Terry and Nicole could also have shifted focus away from resentment and onto actively creating better experiences in their lives.

KEEP IT PEACEFUL

We do not have to assert ourselves in painful or anxiety-producing relationships by becoming fat; instead we can decide to respond to the stresses of the relationship in ways that are benign to ourselves and others. This requires a determined, conscious intent to relinquish weapons and to find a means of dealing peacefully with the other person or of peacefully going our separate way. Finding inner peace, rather than controlling others, should be our focus in choosing our response. It helps if we remember that the usual result of trying to manipulate, control or score against others is that our own unhappiness tends to increase.

When we are determined to use peaceful means, a benign resolution usually presents itself in even the most convoluted of relationships. To be in the proper mindset for this to happen, we can once again rely on spiritual Power. It can be helpful to use the following affirmation:

> *I recognize that there is always a benign way of dealing with other people, benign for me and benign for them. Through the power of the Divine, the perfect, peaceful way of dealing with this relationship is becoming clear now. A peaceful resolution is prevailing, and I give thanks.*

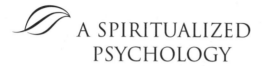

A SPIRITUALIZED PSYCHOLOGY

This chapter has presented you with a significant amount of work to do in order to alter the subconscious motivations that have impelled you to become fat. This work of understanding the meaning and function of your excess weight, and freeing yourself from these subconscious motivations through reliance on spiritual power, will result in a spiritualization of your psychology. Your conscious and subconscious minds will align themselves with your Higher Self and its desire to express the Divine. You will take not only a giant step towards reaching your perfect weight, but also a giant step towards achieving a "Paradise on Earth" mentality. You will stop being at cross purposes with your own Soul and instead will take on its perspective of seeing all the circumstances of your life as opportunities for creating Paradise.

We can find a perfect example of this perspective of the Soul in the life of Jesus, as recounted in St. John's description of Jesus' healing of the man who was blind from birth. In this incident, the disciples ask Jesus whether the man was born blind as punishment for his sins or the sins of his parents. Jesus refuses to blame anyone but instead says that the man is blind "so that the power of God might be manifest in him." He views the man's blindness as an opportunity to create a healing that will express the grace and power of God. Jesus viewed the apparently negative circumstance of the man's blindness from the perspective of a thoroughly spiritualized consciousness that saw in every circumstance the opportunity to express the Divine. This is the perspective from which wonderful changes result.

The spiritualization of your psychology can result in a transformation in your attitude and behavior that will take you far beyond all your previous attempts at change. If you approach the work given in this chapter with an awareness of its spiritualizing impact, you will experience it as an exciting, natural, and joyous pastime. It will take time, but it will not seem time-consuming or tedious. You will become increasingly happy to do it as its powerful effects become manifest in your life.

3

Accessing

Your

Perfect Form

B ESIDES CHANGING YOUR PHILOSOPHY and your psychological motivations, you must also change your body image if you want to reach your perfect weight. Your body image is a crucial component in determining your weight and appearance, since your subconscious mind tends to accept your body image as a blueprint for how it should design your body. If you work with the material presented in Chapters One and Two, you will notice that your image of your body will automatically start shifting away from one that is negative to one that is positive, lighter, and more energetic.

This chapter will present additional suggestions for creating a new body image. It is essential to have an image of your body as trim, fit, attractive, and harmoniously proportioned—not only in order to achieve your perfect weight, but also to maintain it. We frequently regain the weight we have struggled so hard to lose because our new appearance is inconsistent with our old image of ourselves, and this inconsistency results in inner panic and the fear of loss of identity.

I have called this chapter on body image "Accessing Your Perfect Form" because I accept the Neoplatonic concept that we already exist in our perfect form as an idea in Divine Mind, and I believe that we can access the attributes of ourselves as a Divine idea, or ideal form, since these attributes are already intrinsically ours. In creating a new body image we are not inventing anything new but are rather becoming more aware of ourselves as we already are at the highest level of our being. Our efforts to create a new image can rely on the assurance that in doing so we are moving towards our true identity rather than the artificial identity presented by our disguise of fat.

YOUR CURRENT BODY IMAGE

As a starting-point for developing a new body image, it is useful to know what your current image consists of. To find out, write a few paragraphs describing what you look like. When you have finished writing, read through your description to see if it is a balanced one. Does it make mention of those aspects of your appearance that you *like*, as well as those you don't? When we are overweight, we sometimes unduly focus on our "bad" points, never noticing, for example, that we may have beautiful eyes or hands, a graceful walk, or an attractive voice.

In reading through your description, also notice whether you have interpreted some quality of your body as detrimental when it is really a neutral or even beneficial quality. We tend to gravitate towards an unduly negative interpretation of our physical traits if our sense of self-worth is low or we are feeling discouraged. For example, women who are tall and large-boned may view their big frames as clumsy or unfeminine, instead of viewing them neutrally, simply as large frames—or positively, as a source of strength in performing physical tasks or in helping someone who is physically weaker.

REWRITE FOR SELF-ACCEPTANCE

Give some thought to any of your body characteristics that you have failed to appreciate or may have misinterpreted. Then rewrite your description with new awareness, making it a truly realistic portrait of yourself, rather than one that is negatively skewed. When you have finished your rewrite, add to it the final sentence: *I love myself, I accept myself, and I wish myself all the best.*

By performing this writing exercise, you are helping to shift your body image away from one that is dominated by negativity to one that is more balanced. You are also opening yourself to the beneficial influence of self-acceptance. It is paradoxical but true that change comes about more easily when we practice self-acceptance; when we accept ourselves as we are, with no blame or criticism, we are giving ourselves a fresh start to become whatever we want to be. We must remember that being fat is not a crime, no matter how much the media and the fashion industry may imply that it is.

Too often we have hated being fat, or hated ourselves because we are fat. In the Hindu and Jain philosophies of India, we find the profound insight that hatred forges a powerful vibrational bond between us and that which we hate, a bond that keeps us and the object of our hatred firmly attached to each other. We must stop hating our fat if we wish to be free of fat.

Self-acceptance is the antidote to this hatred and liberates us to a world of new possibilities. We must have a complete picture of ourselves rather than just a negative one, and we must accept all of our characteristics without blame, considering them as helpful clues to the world of our inner beliefs.

Keep your rewritten description at hand, since we will be returning to it after you perform the other exercises in this chapter. Right now, having accepted your current self-image in its totality, you are in an excellent position to begin consciously releasing the "fat self" aspect of this image. Your fat self-image must be relinquished before you can successfully create your image anew.

RELEASING STORED EMOTIONS

Our fat self-image is often ingrained in us far more deeply than we realize. The more deeply entrenched our fat self-image is in our minds, the harder it is for us to change our appearance. A fat self-image is both a cause and an effect of being fat; your image of yourself as a fat person grows stronger the more persistent your weight problem is, and this in turn makes your weight problem even more persistent. To break out of this cycle, you must free yourself from the fixed image of yourself as a fat person.

A useful exercise for dissolving your fat self-image is to imagine that the emotions stuck in your body as fat are being released. In Chapter Two, I mentioned that emotions are energy and that emotions which become stuck in the body turn into fat, or stored energy. We often find it very hard to release our anger, fear, resentment, bitterness, etc., even when we consciously want to let go of these destructive feelings. Sometimes even years of therapy are of no avail against the strength and holding power of these emotions.

In dealing with myself and people I have counseled, I have found that altruism can be the key to releasing these persistent emotions. Since emotions are energy, and energy can be changed into another form, we can consciously offer up our stuck emotions to the Higher Power and ask that they be transmuted into a new form of energy that will be helpful to someone else. We can thus sacrifice (literally, "make holy") our negative feelings and put them to good use on someone else's behalf.

For example, you may still feel great anger at a mate who rejected you, even though many years have passed since the relationship ended. You are tired of this anger and would like to be free of it at last. This anger is energy, and someone somewhere could use some energy now, whether that person is a war victim, a hungry child, or a cold and destitute homeless person. You can offer up your anger and send the transmuted energy to someone in need.

VISUALIZATION: OFFERING UP YOUR EXCESS WEIGHT

The following visualization exercise will lead you through this altruistic process. The exercise, which I call "Offering Up Your Excess Weight," can help free you from the grip of the past, bring you great emotional relief, and release you from a fat self-image.

If you are not accustomed to doing visualization exercises, you are in for a treat. Visualization is an excellent tool for change, since your subconscious mind cannot distinguish between what you visualize and what you actually experience in the external world. Inner and outer experience are all one to the subconscious mind and have an equal impact. With practice, anyone can visualize. Before performing this visualization, read through the description a few times to become familiar with it. If you wish, you can record it on a cassette player to play back to yourself.

To begin, be comfortably seated, close your eyes, and relax. Take three deep breaths with long exhalations, so that you feel even more relaxed. With your eyes still closed, raise them slightly. Now visualize a place that is your own special, private place. This place is completely safe for you and is completely under your jurisdiction; no one can come to your place without your permission. This private place can be a beautiful place outdoors, such as a forest or a beach, or a fabulous penthouse apartment, or any other locale that appeals to you.

Notice all that you can about this special place. See what if looks like; observe the colors and details. Hear the natural sounds of water, wind, or birds; or the distant sound of your butler telling the rest of your staff that you cannot be disturbed; or whatever sounds seem appropriate to your place. Feel the floor or ground under your feet. Notice whether you can detect any fragrance in the air. Let the entire ambiance of this private place give you feelings of security and comfort.

Once you are peacefully ensconced in this special place, imagine that here you have access to all the information you need to help change your body image. Raise your closed eyes, and let information come to you about the predominant emotion that is stuck in your body. Is it anger, fear, bitterness, sadness, resentment, frustration, envy, hatred? Ask for this information, and you will know what the emotion is. When you realize what the emotion is, remind yourself that all emotions are energy, and energy can be transmuted from a harmful to a helpful form.

Stretch your arms out in front of you, palms up, and imagine that the emotion is flowing out of your body and into your palms, forming itself into a ball of energy around the size of a basketball. Really feel the emotion, and really feel the energy of the emotion flowing into your hands and from your hands into the ball shape. What color is the ball? Anger and resentment often appear to be fiery red with black edges, and sadness a murky gray, but an emotion may be any color. See the color of your emotion as it forms the ball of emotional energy.

Then raise your arms up in a gesture of offering the colored energy ball up to the Higher Power for transmutation. Say "Almighty, Holy One (or similar words), I offer you this emotion to transmute into a beneficial form. I direct the transmuted energy to go to someone who needs it." See the ball of energy changing color into silver, gold, pure white, or some other color that instills a sense of peace in you, and then see it rising out of your hands and floating way up into the sky. Know that it will go to a person who needs the energy at this time.

Bring your hands back down by your sides, and when you feel ready, slowly open your eyes and come back to normal consciousness. Realize that you have taken a major step in the process of dissolving your fat self-image.

I suggest that you perform this exercise at least once a week until you reach your perfect weight. The predominant stored emotion may vary from week to week, or you may find that the same one comes up several weeks in a row. You can also use this exercise when you are in the grip of a strong current of emotion (rather than a stored one) that you would like to be free of. Using this exercise will afford you the chance to consciously feel and release powerful negative emotions rather than repress them, foster them, or cling to them by automatically storing them in your body.

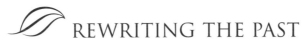 REWRITING THE PAST

Often we have become locked into a fat self-image as a result of the powerful force of memory. Most of us have experienced memorable instances of humiliation connected with being fat. These painful memories of times when we have felt ashamed of being fat perpetuate our old self-image and keep us from accepting a new image as a normal-weight person.

One way to free yourself from the impact of memories of humiliation is to mentally rewrite the history of these painful episodes. Think of a humiliating incident connected with your being fat, and then change the ending of the incident to one that makes you laugh and feel victorious rather than hurt and ashamed. By changing the ending of a negative incident to one that is funny rather than painful, and in which you emerge triumphant rather than humiliated, you will feel cheered up rather than embarrassed whenever you recall the incident. If you re-write the major incidents of humiliation in your life in this way, their sting and thus their hold on your self-image will eventually disappear. In time you will even feel sorry for the people who insulted you, since they were too ignorant to recognize you for the jewel that you are!

Here is an example of this rewriting technique, using a humiliating incident from my own past. This is what actually happened:

> Scene: *Campus of a large midwestern university. I am 18 years old, 5 feet tall, and weigh 185 lb. As I am walking along the tree-lined path to class one day, two young soldiers, about my age, walk past coming from the opposite direction.*

> First soldier: *(looking at me with disgust)* What a dog!

> Second soldier: *(nodding in agreement)* Yeah! I've never seen such a dog!

> *I hurry away from them, feeling totally ashamed and humiliated.*

> Here is the ending as rewritten:

> First soldier: What a dog!

> Second soldier: Yeah! I've never seen such a dog!

> *Suddenly a huge, handsome, hulking giant of a jock emerges from behind the trees. It's my boyfriend,*

"Moose," a fiercely protective type whom no one would ever like to cross. The two soldiers are shocked by his sudden appearance. Moose picks them up by the scruff of the neck.

Moose: You guys have some kind of problem with this lady?

Soldiers: *(trembling)* No, sir!

Moose puts them down roughly, and they run off in abject terror. I feel vindicated, victorious, and very satisfied. Moose puts his arm around me and we go off to spend the rest of the day together.

This revised ending never fails to cheer me up whenever I happen to think about this incident. Moose is a figment of my imagination, but my subconscious mind can't distinguish between imagination and external events, and it accepts this version of the past and releases my old sense of shame connected with this encounter.

You can use this rewriting technique on whatever humiliating weight-related memories still bother you. It is especially important to use it on memories in which you were labeled as being fat by someone in authority or were called names for being fat. For example, when I was in fourth grade I had to visit the doctor because of pains in my arm. I was alone in the examining room waiting for the doctor when I saw my file on his desk. Bored with waiting and naturally curious, I got up from the examining table to look at the file.

The first thing I saw in the file was "OBESE FEMALE CAUCASIAN" written in large letters across the first page. I felt totally mortified. I was a little girl with a good vocabulary, and I knew exactly what the words meant. I am sure that my being labeled in this way by the doctor had a very harmful impact on me and strengthened my already-existent fat self-image.

I have rewritten this incident so that when I open the file I see the words "THIS WONDERFUL CHILD IS DESTINED FOR GREAT THINGS." I always feel happy now when I think of this incident, since it is the rewritten version that comes to mind.

Let your imagination have free rein to transform your painful memories into episodes from which you emerge the winner. You can actually write out a particular experience and its revised ending, as I have done here, or you can perform the exercise mentally. Whichever you choose to do, enjoy the experience of your revised ending to the fullest. By replacing your painful thoughts with thoughts that cheer you, you are liberating yourself from the old and are happily moving forward towards acceptance of a new self-image.

OVERCOMING FEAR OF THINNESS

Our attitude towards thinness may also keep us locked in our fat self-image. Because we tend to think dualistically, many of us think that the only alternative to being fat is to be thin, meaning *really* thin. We view weight in terms of the polarity of fatness and thinness instead of seeing it as a *spectrum of possibilities,* with our particular perfect weight lying somewhere in the spectrum's middle portion. If we think in such a dualistic way, we may subconsciously cling to our fat self-image because of a negative attitude towards thinness.

Thinness is supposedly the ideal of our contemporary culture, and we spend millions of dollars each year in its pursuit, but to many of us thinness nevertheless means vulnerability and weakness. We consider thinness an unprotected, defenseless state of being. We may also equate thinness with skinniness, boniness, gawkiness, or some other negatively perceived quality.

WHAT'S IN A WORD?

What do you think of when you hear the word *thin?* I suggest that you take a minute to free-associate and jot down as many associations as come to you. You will probably be surprised at how negative some of your responses are. When it first occurred to me to do this, I was surprised to see that I associated being thin with having osteoporosis. No wonder I'd had so much difficulty becoming thin! I also free-associated with the word *slim* and found that the major image that came to mind was an old cowhand in a Western movie, not at all the kind of person I'd want to look like!

Words are powerful, so if the words *thin* and *slim* evoke unpleasant associations for you, select a different adjective to describe your desired state. Many people do well using the words *fit* and *trim* instead. You can also remind yourself that the process of losing weight can make you thinner and slimmer without making you "thin" or "slim."

The word *slender* is used in many weight-loss programs; I personally like it because it rhymes with *tender,* and because, according to the dictionary it means "having graceful proportions." To many people, however, *slender* may have connotations of slightness and inconsequentialness; men may also consider it an adjective appropriate only for women. When thinking about how you would look if you lost weight, be sure that the adjectives you use have only pleasant connotations for you.

One adjectival phrase that I've found everyone can relate well to is "normal weight." We all know the difference between excess weight and normal weight, and we all tend to accept "normal weight" as something desirable. "Normal weight" also gives us a sufficient range from which we can choose the weight that is really perfect for our individual frame. It can relieve a lot of pressure from us and make it easier to release our fat self-image if we see our goal as reaching a normal weight rather than becoming "thin" or "slim."

For many of us, "becoming normal-weight" or "changing to perfect weight" may be more helpful terms to use than "losing weight." Ordinarily we connect the words *lose* and *loss* with situations involving missing objects, failure, lack, deprivation, bereavement, and lapse of emotional control. If *loss* and *lose* arouse negative associations in us, we may subconsciously resist our conscious efforts to change our body image in the direction of weight loss.

WILL WE VANISH WITH OUR FAT?

Even when we replace such words as thin, slim, and lose with words that are less threatening to us, we still must face the very real fear that most of us have of decreasing our weight. "Who will I be when I lose 20 lb. [50 lb., 100 lb.] or more?" is a completely valid question. Will I be diminished as a person? Will the intrinsic me disappear? What will remain of me when my current body presentation is so altered? We have become so identified with our fat that at our deepest level we believe that if our fat vanishes, we will vanish too. If we were told that tomorrow morning we would wake up and find ourselves at a normal weight, most of us would feel not joy but fear and panic.

Indeed, a major weight loss can be a frightening proposition. It can be terrifying to look in the mirror and no longer recognize yourself. I can remember actually letting out a scream when I looked in a full-length mirror after losing 95 lb. and didn't recognize myself. Who was that stranger in the glass who had replaced my old reflection?

Sometimes just receiving a compliment on a weight loss can induce a sense of panic in us. People who have lost a great deal of weight will sometimes start feverishly overeating after being complimented, in order to control this panic. Something in the compliment is so at odds with their old self-image that they subconsciously fear they are close to annihilation and believe they must regain weight in order to continue existing.

WE ARE NOT OUR FAT

To overcome our deep-rooted fear of losing weight, it is crucial that we stop identifying with our fat. We are not our excess weight; we created it to express something and to serve some function, but it is not us. To let go of our weight means to alter our appearance, not lose our identity. Our fat is a disguise that we have utilized for understandable reasons and can now set aside. We can appreciate and even love our fat because it has attempted to fulfill our needs, but we must not equate it with our identity.

Our Higher Self is our eternal identity; our identity on earth is that of spiritual beings who are here in order to express the Divine on the physical plane. Balance and harmony are attributes of the Higher Self, and good health and perfect weight are physical expressions of these spiritual qualities. When you manifest your perfect weight, you are not losing your identity but are actually expressing your true identity more accurately.

Every day, look at yourself in the mirror and say, *"You are a spiritual being who has come here to express the Divine on the physical plane."* Talking to yourself in the mirror is an extremely direct and effective way of communicating a message to your subconscious mind. If you remind yourself of your spiritual identity, you will find that your attachment to your fat, and thus to your fat self-image, will melt away. At the same time, your sense of self-worth and deserveability will go skyrocketing. You will lose your fear of weight loss and will be able to accept a new, normal-weight self-image with self-confidence and anticipation.

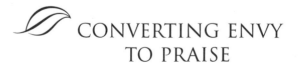

CONVERTING ENVY TO PRAISE

To speed up your liberation from your old self-image, make a conscious effort to relinquish any envy or jealousy you may have of people who are normal-weight or thin. Sometimes we feel envious and resentful when we see someone with a great body or an exceptional figure, or someone who can eat enormous amounts of food and never gain an ounce. In addition to feeling envious, we may even feel condescending towards these people and think that they must be shallow because they haven't suffered as we have suffered by being fat. These feelings are not helpful; if negative feelings arise in you when you encounter someone who is at their perfect weight, your subconscious mind may get the message "perfect weight evokes hostility" and may thus faithfully strive to keep you from ever looking like this person!

Remember that we all face different challenges throughout our lives; these people are "masters" of weight, but they are no doubt facing other challenges that you are not aware of. For all you know, they may even have overcome a weight problem at some earlier point in their lives. I am constantly amazed at the number of people who tell me that at one time in their lives they weighed 75 or 100 lb. more than they do now; it is really amazing how people's appearances can change. You should never simply assume that someone with a beautiful body does not understand what it's like to be overweight.

Instead of feeling resentful and thinking "It's not fair!" when you see someone who has a good shape or is effortlessly thin, train yourself to think *"Good for you! You have mastered your weight, and I know that I can do the same. I want to look more like you. Thank you for inspiring me!"* In this way, your identification with your fat will lessen. Your subconscious mind will get the message that perfect weight is a condition that you find desirable rather than one to which you are hostile. Moreover, the stultifying energy of resentment in your body will be replaced by the free-flowing, enlivening energy of appreciation and praise.

PRACTICING SELF-FORGIVENESS

Self-forgiveness is also essential if we are to relinquish our old self-image. Unless we forgive ourselves, we will be ever mired in the past and confined by our old ways of perception. Often we do not forgive ourselves even when we believe that God forgives us. We block ourselves from accepting the sense of spiritual cleansing and restoration that Divine Mercy always makes available to us. It's as though we tell ourselves, "God may forgive me, but I will never let myself off the hook."

This attitude is cruel, unproductive, and contrary to the nature of the Divine. Be kind to yourself, and let go of whatever feelings of guilt or self-recrimination you may have accumulated over the years. You must consciously practice self-forgiveness as part of a commitment to renouncing self-punishment and to shifting your orientation away from the past.

The following visualization exercise will help you achieve self-forgiveness. Prior to doing it for the first time, I suggest that you spend some time thinking of the things that you have done that you have not forgiven yourself for. You may be immediately aware of many of these, but others may lie below the surface of your conscious mind, long-forgotten though still unforgiven by you.

SELF-EXAMINATION TECHNIQUE

An effective way to proceed with this self-examination is to set a timer for five minutes and then complete the sentence "I feel guilty about————" as many times as endings for the sentence come to mind in the five-minute period. Do this out loud. Then set the timer two more times, and do the same thing with the sentences "I feel inadequate because————" and "I feel angry with myself because————" This simple 15-minute technique will bring to your awareness all the things that you have been holding against yourself and that must be forgiven if you are to get on with your life and with the fulfillment of your Soul's purpose. You cannot express your Higher Self and work towards the creation of Paradise on Earth if you stay locked in your mental cage of nonforgiveness, the jail in which you are jailer and prisoner at the same time.

SELF-FORGIVENESS VISUALIZATION

After completing your self-examination, you can use the following visualization to carry out the self-forgiveness process. As with all the visualizations given in this book, you should read through the description of the visualization a few times to become familiar with it before doing it, or make a recording of it on a cassette player for your personal use. Get into a relaxed state and prepare to wash away all of your unforgiven actions and qualities in the River of Life, whose waters are the waters of forgiveness.

Sit comfortably, close your eyes, and completely relax. Take three deep breaths, with long exhalations so that you feel even more relaxed. With your eyes still closed, raise them slightly and visualize a place outdoors that is your own special private place. See what this place looks like. It's a bright sunny day in spring or summer, so notice the blue sky, the vivid green trees and grass, and the colorful flowers. Hear the sounds of the birds and smell the scent of pine or flowers. Feel the earth below your feet and the gentle breeze as it caresses your face.

Stay for a minute in this special place, feeling more relaxed and secure all the time. Then notice a path leading through the trees. Follow the path, and it will take you to the shores of a beautifully flowing river. Hear the soothing and refreshing sound of the waters flowing. In your visualization, take off your clothes and walk into the river. As the water reaches your knees, you realize that this is a magical river and that the water is flowing through you as well as around you. You know that in this river it is safe to submerge yourself completely and let whatever needs forgiveness to be gently washed away.

Lie down in the river, feeling completely safe, and let the cleansing waters flow over you and through you. Feel all of the feelings of guilt, inadequacy, and anger with yourself dissolve and wash away. The water is washing them gently and surely away. They are safely and completely washed away. You know that you are forgiven, and that you can go on now with a wonderful new stage of your life.

You get up from the river, and return to the shore. Where you left your clothes, you see a beautiful white robe. You put it on and walk back down the path to your special place. When you get there, see that someone has left a beautiful blanket for you to sit on. You sit down on it and are immediately overcome with a sense of gratitude for the wonderful gift of forgiveness that you have been given.

You mentally raise your arms to heaven and mentally say, "Thank you, thank you!" Then, when you are ready, you slowly come back to normal consciousness and open your eyes. You raise your arms to heaven and say out loud, "Thank you, thank you!"

I suggest that you perform this visualization exercise at least once a month. It will have a profound effect on your ability to forgive yourself and to increasingly treat yourself with compassion.

If some of your guilt feelings are due to the fact that you have caused pain or sorrow to others, you can supplement this visualization work by deciding on a method or reparation. Often we cannot atone directly to the people we have hurt, either because they are no longer alive or we are no longer acquainted with them, or because it would be inappropriate for some reason.

We can always make some kind of reparation, however, by praying for their well-being, by making contributions to charity, or by performing some kind of volunteer work that is meaningful to us. This work of reparation is to be undertaken not to punish yourself but rather to contribute to your self-healing as an expression of your self-forgiveness. In the process, you also contribute to others.

Forgiveness is a change of focus, a turning away from past experience in favor of a new direction. As you become more forgiving of yourself, it will be easier for you to forgive those who have hurt you as well. You will feel so much peace and strength arising from self-forgiveness that old hurts and animosities will lose their power over you. You will understand that if you have been nursing old grievances, you have kept alive the injuries that were done to you and have inflicted them on yourself all over again. Holding on to them has kept you chained to the past instead of moving forward. You will realize that for your own sake, it is better to forgive and move on.

TREATING YOUR BODY AS YOUR BELOVED CHILD

When we truly forgive ourselves, we create a new, loving relationship with our body unlike anything we have had in the past. Our body is our own creation, and by practicing self-forgiveness we naturally come to love our body as we would a beloved child. This is a responsible kind of love; in addition to feeling affection and appreciation for our body, we want to give it everything it needs to be · healthy and happy. We want to separate it as much as possible from influences that are detrimental to its well-being.

When we treat our body as our beloved child, we see to it that it has the right type and amount of food, rest, exercise, fun, education, and interaction with others. We give it scope to develop its talents, and we indulge it whenever we can, as long as this indulgence will not prove harmful to it.

The more we practice self-forgiveness, the more we love our body; and the more we love our body, the more self-forgiveness we feel. By consciously treating your body as your beloved child, you can expedite the self-forgiveness process.

EXAMINE YOUR DAILY ROUTINE

You can begin to cultivate this new attitude towards your body right away. Begin by considering your daily routine and checking your body's reactions to your habitual daily patterns.

To start with, how many hours of sleep do you get at night, and in which time period do you get them? If you consider yourself a night owl and think that staying up late is your natural pattern, ask yourself how your body is responding to this pattern. Is it thriving, as you would wish if it were your beloved child? Or does it feel jittery, irritable, and unfocused in the daytime? If you have gotten into the habit of not getting up till late in the morning, does your body feel as energetic as it did when you used to rise earlier, or does it feel listless and groggy?

How would your body feel if you went to bed an hour earlier than you do now? Experiment in order to find the amount of sleep and the sleeping schedule that are best for your body. It is no exaggeration to state that the quality of your sleep determines the quality of your waking life; peaceful days can only come from restful nights! You will know that your body is receiving what it needs when you can wake up naturally, without an alarm clock, feeling totally refreshed and eager to face the day.

YOUR BODY LOVES EXERCISE

Most of us follow a very sedentary lifestyle that the body was not designed for. You can experiment to see how your body would feel if you were to increase the amount of time you spend walking or exercising and decrease the amount of time you spend driving or watching television. When the body is sedentary too much of the time, it becomes listless and irritable; it feels heavy, stuck, and incapable of initiating anything new. The body is composed of energy, and as an energetic being it must express its fundamental quality of being in motion in order to thrive. A daily routine that is too sedentary creates intense frustration in the body.

Your body loves to exercise; exercise relieves stress, gives tone to the body, and improves all body functions. Brisk walking is an excellent form of exercise that requires no special skill and costs nothing in fees or equipment. If your lifestyle is too sedentary, try to incorporate at least half an hour a day of brisk walking into your schedule. If you can work a full hour a day of brisk walking into your schedule, you will experience a really remarkable change in your shape and in your body's sense of well-being.

Tai Chi, Chi Kung (Qi Gong), and other Eastern forms of exercise are greatly conducive to the body's health and are gentle enough to be done even by those who are extremely out of shape. Often when we are very fat we feel too awkward to join an exercise class. Now, luckily, many excellent videos exist so that we can learn these health-giving exercises in the privacy of our homes. These Eastern exercises heal our inner organs and strengthen our life force so that our entire physiology can return to optimum functioning.

Exercises for spot reducing are also very helpful and can be a great source of encouragement since they can change certain body contours so quickly. Some of the best exercise books for slimming your waist, thighs, buttocks, etc., are those very inexpensive little booklets frequently found near the check-out in supermarkets. These booklets cost next to nothing but provide invaluable information for reducing specific areas of your body. Become committed to learning about various types of exercise and to providing your body with exercise on a regular basis.

CHECK YOUR DIET

Check to see how your eating and drinking habits are affecting your body. Does your body feel sluggish and bloated after meals, because you are eating too much, too quickly, or the wrong food? Does it feel jittery from too much coffee and tea, hyper from soft drinks, or spaced out from alcohol?

While you may feel a temporary boost from sugar, junk food, caffeine, and alcohol, how does your body feel after this temporary stimulation has passed? Notice whether these temporary highs are followed in a couple of hours by cravings for more of these false stimulants. If they are, it is a sign that your body has felt a down after the high and is trying misguidedly to correct the down through more stimulation.

When you love your body, you want it to be completely healthy and free from the addictive cycle of false stimulation and craving. You want it to always feel calm, comfortable, and strong. By viewing your body as your beloved child, you will become increasingly interested in providing your body with food and drink that nourishes it and allows it to thrive. You will want to know exactly what is in your food and drink and what effects these ingredients will have on your body.

It is a good idea to get in the habit of noticing how your body feels at a given moment. Train yourself to take note of your body's sensations and emotions; these may differ from your own conscious desires and may require other priorities. Give your body a break if you note that it feels too full to eat any more, too tired to work any more, or too wired to watch any more TV.

EXPERIENCE YOUR EMOTIONS CONSCIOUSLY

Emotions often register in the body before we experience them in our consciousness. By observing your body closely, you can discern the emotions that are present in your body though submerged below the level of your conscious awareness. For example, notice how you are carrying yourself. Are your hands clenched, which is a sign of anxiety, or are your shoulders hunched up in tension? Has your skin broken out, which is a sign of stress? Does your stomach or any other organ feel upset?

Clothing is an extension of the body; are you wearing much darker clothing or much baggier clothing than usual? Such clothing changes can be indications of feelings of sadness or shame. Look for these body clues and ask yourself what is underlying them. If your beloved child were showing these signs of inner distress, you would surely want to know more about what was happening. Allow the emotions of fear, anger, shame, etc., represented by your body clues to come into your conscious awareness. We must experience our emotions consciously if we are to keep them from being stuck in the body.

For good health, we must feel our negative emotions rather than suppress them, and release them rather than hold on to them. There are many harmless ways to release our emotions; we can cry, we can yell, we can hold imaginary conversations with the people we are angry at. We can offer up our emotions to be transmuted, as in the exercise given earlier in this chapter.

Sometimes emotions can be expressed and released by the simplest kind of verbalization, such as simply saying out loud "I feel sad," "I feel angry," etc. Better yet, you can say "I feel sad about ... " or "I feel mad because ... " and fully verbalize the entire situation that is bothering you. No one else needs to be present; the important thing is to allow yourself to feel the emotion and to release it by expressing it verbally. Do this out of concern for your body's well-being.

When we treat our body with this tender concern, observing its reactions and making an effort to release these sensations and emotions, we feel flooded with love for ourselves and vibrant with new potential. Like a sunflower turning to the sun, we move effortlessly into a new mindset that is free of the past and open to creating a new body image.

TRANSCENDING THE ISSUE OF DESERVING

Deserving is often a major issue in our inability to give up our fat self-image. For numerous reasons we may believe that we don't deserve to be a normal weight or to have the freedom from suffering that would result if our weight were normal. Feelings of unworthiness tend to run very deeply in most of us and often lurk beneath our fears of losing weight. We may very genuinely fear that we will disappear if we lose weight; we may worry that our best friend will become jealous of us, that our spouse will feel threatened by our heightened attractiveness, or that our lecherous boss will start to harass us. Sometimes, though, as real as these fears are, they may function as a distraction from the main issue that is holding us back, which is our belief that we do not deserve to be a normal weight.

Your subconscious mind can overcome its conviction that you are undeserving, if you faithfully do the work suggested in this book and if you get in the habit of noticing and interrupting your self-critical thoughts whenever they arise. Moreover, the entire question of deserving can become moot if you love your body as if it were your beloved child. When acting as a loving parent to a child, you would never raise the question of whether your child "deserved" the good things you were giving it; you would give them not because of any deserving on the child's part but simply because it is your child and you love it. Where enough love is present, deserveability is transcended and becomes a non-issue.

When we no longer have to "deserve" to be a normal weight, we can move rapidly forward into weight loss based on a new self-image independent of the constraints of the past. Eliminating the question of deserveability also removes the main obstacle to our accepting a prime source of help in losing weight—the help that is available to us through the power of prayer.

PRAY—WITH CONFIDENCE

Many of us never consider praying about our weight problem, no matter how much unhappiness our excess weight may be causing us. We think that prayer should be reserved for "serious" problems, such as illness, job loss, natural disasters, etc. Weight seems too trivial or frivolous a subject for prayer. Indeed, many people find it hard to ever pray for anything for themselves, even though they may regularly pray for other people.

Our reluctance to pray for ourselves in general, or to pray about our weight, comes from our deep-rooted feelings of unworthiness. We believe that we do not deserve to have what we want, or even to ask for it. However, even if we shy away from praying for ourselves in the traditional way because of these feelings of unworthiness, we can benefit from the prayer power inherent in affirmations.

Affirmations based on spiritual power, such as those given in Chapter Two, are a form of prayer in which, by aligning ourselves with the Divine, we allow an already perfect Divine Reality to become manifest on the physical plane. Traditional, petitionary prayer also has its place, though; it is natural for human beings to say "Help me" to the Higher Power when in distress, and we should cultivate the habit of praying for help with our weight.

As we grow in love for our body, we will find that any reluctance we may have about praying for perfect weight will be eliminated. Since deserving will no longer be an issue, we will feel free to ask for exactly what we want.

PRAYER A CHANGE OF MIND

Our prayers can be answered only if our consciousness is ready to receive what we are asking for. Our consciousness is like a gateway between heaven and earth; the gateway must be unblocked if we are to receive the heavenly gifts that await us. Affirmations, which can also be called affirmative prayer, change our consciousness by aligning us with the already existent perfection of the Spirit. Petitionary prayer should also seek to change our consciousness. The New Testament writers frequently mention the need for metanoia, which in earlier translations from the Greek was translated as "repentance," but actually means "change of mind." The success of our prayers will be blocked if we do not undergo this change of consciousness. Our consciousness must become a clear gateway, free of the obstacles of fear, guilt, self-criticism, resentment, and anger at ourselves and others.

When we pray in the petitionary way, therefore, it is helpful not only to ask for what we want but also to *ask that our consciousness be changed* to make what we want possible. If you choose to pray about your weight, a good prayer is *"Please let my consciousness be changed so that I can reach my goal weight."* When you pray in this way, you open yourself to a strong influx of grace, or assistance from the Higher Power, because you have taken a first step towards clearing the gateway. Pray with confidence, knowing that you are increasingly committed to self-love, self-forgiveness, and the relinquishing of hostile feelings towards others. You can be assured that your old habits of criticizing yourself and judging others will be replaced by the self-acceptance and understanding that make it possible for you to receive the good you desire.

DISCONNECTING FROM SELF-CRITICISM

You can actively increase self-acceptance by stopping the flow of self-criticism whenever it arises in your mind. In the past, this flow may have been so automatic that you were unaware of it. As your love for your body increases, you will be much more alert to negative self-talk and will be able to shut it off as soon as it starts up.

Self-criticism is usually a highly exaggerated response to an incident that has undermined our self-confidence in some way. For example, if we were not hired for a job we wanted, we may respond with the self-critical and self-deprecating thoughts "I'm a failure," "I never get what I want," or "I'll probably never work again." If we gain weight, we may think "I'll never lose weight," "I'm a fat pig," etc. To combat such judgmental, self-defeating thoughts, we should point out to ourselves the finite meaning of these incidents and *note how exaggerated our response has been.* We can tell ourselves that not getting a job means that we did not get the job—not that our whole life is a failure. Similarly gaining weight means that *we have gained weight* (period)—not that we will never lose weight or that we are somehow subhuman because we have gained weight.

USING MENTAL IMAGERY

In addition to turning off the flow of self-criticism by noticing its exaggerated quality, we can turn it off by using mental imagery. When you catch yourself indulging in self-criticism, imagine yourself pulling the plug on a machine, pressing the "delete" key on a computer, or turning off a cassette- or CD-player. Tell yourself "I'm a changed character now, and I'm disconnecting from self-criticism." If you grew up with records rather than cassettes and CDs, it can be very powerful to imagine yourself lifting the needle of a record player from a stuck groove in a record. This simple image provides a strong statement to your subconscious that you are getting out of the groove of old patterns of self-criticism and that you refuse to be stuck in them any longer.

CUTTING THE GORDIAN KNOT

Another helpful image for ending negative self-talk is that of cutting the Gordian knot. If you remember, Alexander the Great was told that whoever managed to unravel the Gordian knot would someday rule the world. Instead of attempting to unravel the massively tangled knot, Alexander simply cut through it with his sword. When you catch yourself having thoughts that berate and belittle yourself, imagine yourself cutting through the Gordian knot of self-criticism with the powerful sword of change.

EXPRESSING GRATITUDE

Expressing gratitude towards your body is another way to foster self-acceptance and break the habit of self-criticism. There are so many reasons that we should be grateful to our bodies; they provide us with so many ways in which to express ourselves and to enjoy the pleasures of the earth plane. Think about the things that you are especially grateful to your body for. Then write out a list of all of your favorite bodily abilities and experiences. Your list might include a wonderful sexual relationship, delicious food, swimming, musical talent, the feel of your favorite cotton shirt, or whatever other pleasures you feel grateful for.

After you have finished writing, look at yourself in the mirror and say, *"I am grateful to you, my body, for*————*"* and read your list out loud. This exercise may sound fanciful, but it is actually a potent way of re-enforcing your love for your body and communicating your gratitude to it.

⟋ EXPERIENCING JOY

One of the most loving things that you can do for your body is to *provide it with more joy.* Joy is the feeling of intense happiness that wells up from inside us when we experience something that is deeply meaningful to us at the soul level. When we are in a condition of joy, happiness permeates every cell of our body. We feel buoyant and blissful from the inside out.

Joy has such a unique quality that most of us can easily recall the most joyful occasions of our lives. These may include our wedding day, the birth of a child, the completion of a significant project, our arrival at a place we have always wanted to visit, the news of a friend's recovery from illness, etc. Joy arises in us when our prayers have been answered or our most heartfelt desires have been fulfilled. Sometimes joy overtakes us quite unexpectedly; we are working at something we love to do, or we read something very inspiring, or we suddenly think about someone we love, and suddenly we are flooded with joy.

When we feel joy, our entire body is soothed, strengthened, and exalted. Joy is a magical balm that lets us heal and develop through delight rather than through any effort.

EXERCISE FOR JOY

More and more joy will tend to come into our lives as we grow in self-forgiveness and acceptance of ourselves. We can also provide ourselves with joy whenever we want to by practicing the following exercise:

> Sit comfortably, with your eyes closed and your hands placed on your thighs, palms up. Relax. Let the relaxation flow down your head and into your neck, your shoulders, arms, midsection, hands, belly area, thighs and calves, and into your feet. Feel deeply and completely relaxed.

Now, in your relaxed state think of something that makes you feel joyful. It can be a memory of a particular occasion, the thought of a particular person, or any other thought that makes you feel joyful. *Really feel the joy;* allow it to intensify as much as possible.

Then sense that the feeling of joy is pervading every part of your body; you are being thoroughly and completely filled with joy. When your body is filled with joy, extend the feeling of joy about 3 inches out from your body, so that your body is surrounded by the 3-inch field of joy. You can visualize the joy around your body as golden light, or you can simply feel that it is there around you.

Thoroughly enjoy the experience of having the 3-inch projection of joy around you. After you have enjoyed it for as long as you wish, allow the joy from the 3-inch field to gently soak back into your body and blend with the joy that is within your body. Realize that this experience of joy will lead to even more joy in your life. Then slowly open your eyes and come back to normal consciousness.

Perform this exercise frequently. By practicing it, you are nourishing your body with what it really wants. Your body will respond by becoming happier and healthier, and your mind will become more lucid and inspired.

When you feel joy, you are experiencing Paradise on Earth. The more often you feel it, the more obvious it will become to you that Paradise is your natural state. You will understand at your cellular level that it is possible to live in a constantly joyful, Paradise-like consciousness.

We will discuss more about experiencing Paradise on Earth in Chapter Five. For now, start practicing this exercise as part of the work of dissolving your fat self-image, and it will quickly prepare you to embrace a new self-image that is far more conducive to joy.

SELECTING YOUR
NEW SELF-IMAGE

After performing all of the exercises given thus far, you will be in the right state of mind for creating a new self-image. The work of creation begins with composing a description of yourself as you would like to be. To decide how you would like to look, return to the revised description of your current appearance that you wrote at the start of this chapter. That description was a realistic portrait of how you look right now and included all aspects of your appearance whether you liked them or not.

The description that you are going to write of how you want to look will include only elements that you like. How exactly do you want to look? Select from your revised current description those characteristics that you like and that you want to retain in the future. Then think seriously about *new* characteristics that you would like to have, among them your perfect weight and shape. *You must have a very clear picture of how you want to look* in order to create a new self-image and achieve its expression.

"TRY ON" A PERFECT-WEIGHT BODY

If you have been overweight for quite some time or for as long as you can remember, it may be hard to imagine what you would look like at your perfect weight or anywhere within a normal-weight range. If this is the case, try to find an example by noticing people who have a similar build (height and bone structure) to yours but who are normal-weight. Then imagine yourself with a body like theirs. Mentally try it on—what does it look like? Can you clearly see yourself in such a body? Keep visualizing yourself with a normal-weight or perfect-weight body until the image becomes familiar to you and you can view it with no feelings of strangeness or trepidation.

If you were formerly a normal weight, it can be helpful to find a photo of yourself at that weight and keep it where you can see it several times a day. When you look at the photo, feel happy at the thought that you are returning to a normal weight and are even going to reach your perfect weight. Tell the image of yourself in the photo "We're going to be thin again. I can do it!" *Remember what it felt like* to be trim and free of excess poundage.

BE TRUE TO YOUR TYPE

When you are deciding how you want to look, be true to your type. If you are a six-foot-tall female with broad shoulders, do not try to look petite! If you are very short, do not yearn to be tall and graceful! You can be short and graceful, and very happy. I am addressing these cautions especially to women since women are under so much pressure to conform to artificial standards of beauty, but men must be warned also. If you are a man with a naturally stocky build, you can become trim, but your frame will not become less wide, and it is counterproductive to wish for a long, lean look; wide is fine.

The point is not for all of us to look the same, but for us to express our physical type in its most perfect form, keeping in mind that by perfection we mean our own individual standard of ease and harmonious proportion.

Sometimes we can get a very clear image of how we want our body to look, except for one particular feature. I once knew a woman named Maureen (not her real name) who had always had extremely large thighs. Although she lost a great deal of weight, her thighs remained disproportionately fat. Maureen couldn't even begin to imagine what it would be like to have normal-sized thighs. She prayed for help in creating a new image of her thighs.

Shortly thereafter she was skimming through a mail-order catalogue that featured the company's own staff as models. In the catalogue Maureen came across an ad featuring a woman in a bathing suit who was Maureen's age

(40's) and had her general build, but who had normal-sized thighs. Since the woman in the ad was not a professional model, it was easy for Maureen to identify with her.

From that time on, Maureen could picture herself with smaller thighs. She would frequently sit down, close her eyes, and imagine herself as she would look with normal-weight thighs. After a short time, her thighs became much more proportionate to her body.

If you have trouble picturing a particular aspect of yourself at a normal weight, look for a person around you or in an advertisement to serve as an example. You can pray for the right example to come to your attention.

SELECT YOUR PERFECT WEIGHT

When deciding how much you would like to weigh, be sure you select the weight that is perfect for you, individually. If you have no idea what this weight should be, you can consult height/weight charts in standard diet books, or better yet, find out how much the person you are using as an example weighs. If someone seems like a good example to you, it will be much more useful to base your weight on theirs rather than to select your weight from charts in books. Such charts are often based on unreal standards and give no consideration to many cultural groups' preferences for weights that are higher than those dictated by the film and fashion industries.

COMPOSE A NEW SELF-PORTRAIT

When you have a clear idea of how you want to look, write a new physical description of yourself. In addition to this physical description, describe all the personality traits, talents, and skills that you would like to have. Also describe your ideal lifestyle, portraying yourself performing work you love and other activities you enjoy, surrounded by people who love and support you. Describe your ideal surroundings and possessions. Let your imagination soar.

Now that you realize that you are a spiritual being who has access to Divine resources, and whose nature it is to express the Divine, the opportunity to have the kind of life you want is far more available to you than when your concept of yourself was more limited. Compose a new self-portrait that shows you at your happiest and most fulfilled. This new image of yourself should reflect your true identity as a powerful, healthy, attractive, prosperous, loving, and well-balanced being. It should be completely consistent with your Soul's purpose of creating Paradise on Earth.

Write the new description of yourself entirely in the present, portraying yourself as though you already possessed all the qualities you desire. For example, if you wish to weigh 140 lb., write "I weigh 140 lb." even if you now actually weigh 195. The fact is that at your Soul level you already have everything that you want; your Higher Self is already perfect, and by creating your new self-image in the present tense you are acknowledging this perfection and directing it to appear in your life. *You are reclaiming your true identity* and drawing up a blueprint for manifesting Paradise in all aspects of your life. Give your creative impulses full sway; let your Paradise be exactly as you would like!

Creating this new self-portrait marks the birth of a new self-image and in addition can mark the start of a new, conscious exercise of your creativity in keeping with your purpose in incarnating on the physical plane. Your new self-portrait also represents your goal. Read your self-portrait every day in order to establish your new image deeply within your subconscious mind. Your subconscious will accept this image as a command and will loyally work to create the body changes and other types of transformation that you have envisioned.

VISUALIZING YOUR PERFECT WEIGHT

In addition to reading your new description of yourself every day, it is important to actively visualize how you will look when you reach your perfect weight. I suggest that you read your new self-portrait every morning and set aside a few minutes for visualization every evening.

In your visualization, you should see yourself at your perfect weight and then see yourself in various scenes that show you enjoying the benefits of perfect weight. To give some simple examples, you could see yourself happily shopping for new, smaller-sized clothes; running quickly up the stairs instead of having to stop along the way; and being complimented on how wonderful you look—and graciously accepting the compliment.

Take some time to think out these scenes. You might want your scenes to focus on the increased ease and enjoyment of everyday activities that you will experience when you are at your perfect weight, or you might want to focus on new activities that will be open to you as a result of your weight loss.

When you have your scenes in mind, write them out. Writing gives you a chance to fill in many of the details of the scene. Let the scenes contain many elements that appeal to your five senses.

You only need to write the scenes out once, but you should visualize them every evening until you reach your perfect weight. Prior to visualizing, get yourself comfortably seated with your eyes closed and relax yourself. Then lift up your closed eyes as if looking up at a movie screen, and see before you an image of yourself at your perfect weight. *Notice how perfectly proportioned you are, and how wonderful you look.* Then see your first scene, enjoying it for a minute or so; switch to your second scene, enjoying it for about a minute; and finally, do the same with your third scene. Then slowly open your eyes and return to normal consciousness.

When you perform this visualization exercise, do it with the intention of creating these scenes in your everyday experience and with faith that your intention will be fulfilled. This visualization process will only take a few minutes, but its impact will be profound.

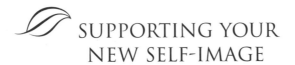

SUPPORTING YOUR NEW SELF-IMAGE

To help support your new self-image, start planning for your future as a perfect-weight person. Begin by going to a department store to look at clothes in the size that you would like to be. It's important to do this so that smaller sizes will not seem foreign or frightening to you when the time comes to wear them. Don't buy the smaller sizes now, but simply get used to looking at them and accepting them as something familiar.

NEW ACTIVITIES

Give some thought to becoming involved in new activities, since there will be more time, energy, and opportunity available to you once you are no longer hindered or preoccupied by the problems of being overweight. Plan ahead, so that you will not feel disoriented by your new-found freedom. Start thinking about dating, if your weight has kept you from doing this, or about going to the beach, taking up a sport, traveling, joining a social group, or anything else you may have been interested in but felt awkward about pursuing because of your weight.

Remind yourself that you do not have to do any of these things, but that you are prepared to have these additional options available to yourself. As part of this preparation, you can send away for travel brochures, get information on health club memberships, etc.

BE PREPARED FOR REACTIONS

Also plan for dealing with the reactions of your friends and family to your new self-image. For example, if your best friend is also overweight, think about how your friend will react when you reach your perfect weight. Will your friend be happy for your success, or jealous and hostile? Will your mate be proud of your accomplishment, or will he or she feel threatened by your new look? Think realistically about any reactions that might occur, and if you foresee difficulties, add to your visualizations a scene in which your friend or mate warmly congratulates you on reaching your goal and tells you how proud they are of your accomplishment.

Frequently affirm:

"Through the power of the Most High, everyone who is important to me helps and encourages me to achieve my perfect weight."

Realize that any fears you may have about your family and friends' reactions may be a projection of your own fears about changing your appearance, and resolve not to let fear hold you back from your good.

You can also support your new self-image by establishing in your mind that success is your pattern. Whenever you accomplish anything that you set out to do, remind yourself that you have succeeded in meeting your goal. In addition, recount to yourself at the end of the day your accomplishments of the day, such as getting the laundry done, spending needed time on family responsibilities, making substantial progress on a project at work, etc.

If you get in the habit of noticing your successes and accomplishments, your subconscious mind will conclude that you are a competent and efficient person who successfully does whatever he or she intends to do, and you will have the full support of your subconscious mind in making a successful switch to your new self-image and your perfect weight.

ALIGNING YOURSELF WITH YOUR PERFECT FORM

I would like to close this chapter with a quick and extremely powerful technique for accepting your new body image and allowing it to manifest quickly in your experience.

Earlier I mentioned the Neoplatonic belief that we already exist in our ideal form as an idea in Divine Mind; I have referred throughout this book to the Higher Self, a contemporary term for this spiritual essence of ourselves which is already perfect in every way and which comprises our true identity.

In this exercise, we will visualize our ideal form and imagine it existing on a higher plane simultaneously with our physical existence on the earth plane. We will align our physical self with our ideal form and by such alignment evoke its perfection into our own bodily experience.

THE ALIGNMENT TECHNIQUE

To begin, get a very clear image in your mind of your ideal form. (Having composed your new self-image, this should be easy to do.) Your ideal form represents you in your most perfect state; see it as being radiantly attractive and having a shape that is fit, trim, and in perfect proportion. Let everything about your ideal form reflect balance, grace, and strength.

Since we are concentrating here on form rather than face, see your ideal form from a rear view. Notice how perfect its weight is for the size of its bones; how harmoniously proportioned it is. Imagine that your ideal form, seen from the rear, is positioned in the air several feet above your head (representing its existence on a higher plane) and about three feet in front of you.

Next move forward and stand directly under where you have imagined your ideal form to be. Stand in complete alignment with your ideal form, facing in the same direction that it is facing. Visualize your ideal form very clearly as you stand below it and say out loud, *"I align myself with my ideal form. As above, so below."* Then, with a feeling of gratitude, go about your everyday activities.

This technique only takes a minute or so, but it is extraordinarily powerful. The technique was inspired by my reading many years ago about certain Renaissance philosophers who held the Neoplatonic view that many levels of reality exist, emanating from the One in a hierarchy of higher and lower levels. These philosophers were preoccupied with understanding correspondences among the various levels of existence and with drawing down and utilizing the energies of the higher levels.

"As above, so below" is the ancient Hermetic formula that acknowledges the influence of the higher realms over the earthly plane and that can serve as an affirmation for calling down this influence. It occurred to me that the ideal form, or pattern of our existence at the highest level, could provide the perfect influence to facilitate weight loss, especially when achieving perfect weight is seen not as an arbitrary challenge but as a desire to express the Soul's innate perfection and artistic mastery.

I realized that standing under the ideal form and aligning oneself with it would make a very graphic statement of receptivity to its influence. I have experienced great benefit from this exercise, and I invite you to try it at least twice a week. It will confirm you in your new self-image and speed up your weight loss accordingly.

As your new self-image grows stronger in your consciousness, new thought patterns will develop within you to free yourself for a more balanced and harmonious way of life. Your food cravings will become more moderate, and your food choices will become more discriminating. Overeating will no longer be a problem for you. You will be able to develop a perfect relationship with food, which brings us to the subject of our next chapter.

4

Approaching

Food

with Reverence

I HAVE SAVED OUR DISCUSSION OF FOOD till the latter part of this book because food is not our main problem, no matter how obsessed we are with it nor how central a place eating and worrying about food may occupy in our daily lives. Our problem lies primarily in our negative attitude towards being incarnated in the physical world, and secondarily in our psychological motivations and self-image. Food is just the means we have used to become fat so that these innermost issues can be expressed externally.

When we do not understand that we have been using food to express our inner concerns, we remain trapped in a highly emotional and destructive relationship with it. We do not want to be fat, but we cannot resist the very foods that make us that way. *We love food—and we hate it.* We feel dissatisfied unless we eat inordinately, and at the same time we despise ourselves for not being able to stop. Food lures us and terrifies us; it is the object of our desire yet a source of intense self-reproach and self-hatred.

Despite our misuse of food, food is not our enemy. Food is a source of life-force energy that we cannot do without. It is a divine gift meant to nourish, sustain, and beautify us. If you do the work suggested in the previous chapters, you will find that your love-hate relationship with food will automatically start to give way to a balanced appreciation of food and a sense of partnership with food in creating your ideal body. This chapter will provide additional suggestions for approaching food with the reverence it deserves and on eating responsibly in accordance with this reverence.

✍ SELECTING OUR FOOD

There are many different diets that have been used success-fully to decrease weight and improve the quality and flow of life-force energy. Deciding what to eat is an individual choice that must take into account your particular body type and your body's responses to various kinds of food.

Some people thrive and lose weight on high-protein diets that focus on meat and cheese, while others do the same on grain-based diets that also include vegetables and fish. Some people do well by counting calories, while others do well by counting carbohydrates or by following principles of food combining in which starches and pro-teins are never eaten at the same meal. Omnivores, carni-vores, vegetarians, vegans, macrobiotics enthusiasts, and raw-foods devotees have all managed to lose weight and be healthy.

Libraries and bookstores are full of information on diet and nutrition, and it can be fun to read up on various theo-ries and decide which ones make sense to you and are com-patible with your personal preferences. The more knowl-edgeable you become about nutrition, including the role of vitamins and other nutritional supplements, the better. It can also be helpful to review any weight-loss information and diet suggestions that have aided you in the past.

It is important to adopt a way of eating that is good for your individual body and that you feel psychologically comfortable with. Only you can choose the way of eating that is best for you. Your diet should be safe, healthy, and appealing enough so that you can follow it indefinitely: in fact, you should think of it as a "foodstyle" (like a lifestyle) rather than a diet, since the word *diet* so often connotes a quick fix that would be harmful or impossible to sustain in the long run.

MY OWN FOODSTYLE

As you work with changing your philosophy, psychology, and body image, you will naturally be drawn to the foodstyle that is best for you. For your consideration, I would like to share with you my own foodstyle, which has helped me and many others, and which people find they can comfortably follow without feeling deprived. This foodstyle is not the only way, but it is a way that I have usually found to be effective.

My foodstyle is based on a desire for high-quality life force and a resulting emphasis on the purity, naturalness, and nutritional value of foods. Food signifies many things to many people; we can see it as a means of fueling our bodies, of experiencing delicious taste sensations, of providing ourselves with love, comfort, and gratification, or even of venting our aggression and symbolically devouring the circumstances of our lives that make us unhappy.

We can switch our orientation away from these common meanings of food, however, and instead focus on food as a source of life-force energy that produces our physical bodies and affects all aspects of our lives. When we change our orientation this way and revere food as a source of life force, we naturally desire those high life-force foods that make us more alive and free. It becomes easy to avoid addictive foods that provide us with temporary gratification at a tremendous cost to our health and well-being.

BASIC GUIDELINES

The following are the basic guidelines for food selection that comprise my foodstyle:

1. *As much as possible, choose foods that are fresh, wholesome, and uncontaminated by pesticides, additives, or preservatives.* When possible, go organic. It is becoming easier all the time to find organically grown grains, beans, vegetables, and fruits, as well as meat, poultry, fish, eggs and dairy

products from naturally raised sources. Once available only at health food stores, many of these foods that are free of harmful chemicals are available at ordinary supermarkets.

Make an effort to buy pure foods, even if you have to go out of your way to do so or have to spend more money than usual. If organically grown fruits and vegetables are not available in your area, at least try to shop at local farmers' markets or farmstands instead of supermarkets, so that your purchases will be fresh and untreated with the extra chemicals needed to ensure long shelf life during transit from farms to distant supermarkets. Giving your body wholesome food is the best investment you can make and is well worth the extra cost or the extra time involved in obtaining it.

If you are shopping for canned, frozen, or other packaged foods, read the labels carefully and don't buy any that contain monosodium glutamate, food dyes, chemical sweeteners, or other chemical additives and preservatives. This includes most commercially prepared desserts, sodas, diet soft drinks, cold cuts, hot dogs, and smoked meats. Smoked foods, even those without extra preservatives, should be eaten only rarely since they are suspected of being carcinogenic. The labels will tell you the number of calories you are consuming as well as alert you to additives in the food.

Always know exactly what you are ingesting. The human body was not designed to eat chemicals, and our contemporary diet, which is so extremely heavily laden with chemicals, has had a disastrous effect not only on our physical and mental health but also on our weight. Food dyes make many people jittery and prone to binges of nervous eating. The drugs that are given to commercially raised livestock and poultry to increase their appetite and speed up their weight gain have the same effect on us as on these animals when we eat these meats. I am convinced that chemicals in our food (not to mention in our drinking supply) are responsible to a very significant extent for the fact that so many of us suffer from suppressed or inadequate metabolism.

Resolve now to free your body as much as possible from the insidious influence of chemicals and drugs in food. I am not suggesting that you stop eating meat from the supermarket or that you adopt a rigid insistence on purity in food that would confine you to food from organically grown or naturally raised sources. I live in New York City, where we have restaurants on every block, and I eat out frequently and enjoy it. I do suggest, however, that you make it a general practice to opt for purity and freshness in food.

At this point I would like to add that recreational drugs must also be avoided. These drugs tend to do great damage to your aura as well as to your body, even if the consequences are not immediately evident to you. If you are taking these drugs now and would like to break the habit, please find a good acupuncturist who can help your body free itself from this addiction and set itself on the path to balance again.

2. *Avoid "partial" foods as much as possible.* Partial foods are foods that have been so refined or processed that they consist of empty calories providing little nutritional value. Refined sugar and white flour are the two partial foods that dominate the standard diet. These foods are so incomplete that they increase our hunger rather than satisfy it.

Foods containing white sugar, such as candy, soft drinks, cookies, doughnuts, pastries, and other desserts should be restricted to special occasions or avoided completely. Once you begin to read labels carefully, you will realize that white sugar is to be found not only in these obviously sweetened foods, but also in foods where you would least expect it, such as in canned vegetables, soups, and other packaged foods. Search for sugar-free alternatives to these products.

Refined sugar stimulates the appetite, destroys vitamins, and sabotages metabolism; it makes you hungrier
for more food and especially for more sugar! If you are
accustomed to eating a breakfast cereal that has refined
sugar in it, try a type that has no added sugar and see how
much less hungry you feel throughout the day. You will
also feel much calmer, since refined sugar is a major
source of irritability, nervousness, mood swings, and
other forms of emotional and physical imbalance.

You can wean yourself off sugar by replacing the sweets
in your diet with cookies and other treats from the health-
food or grocery store that are sweetened with fruit juice,
barley malt, or brown rice sweetener. These desserts are
delicious but much less addictive than sugar-sweetened
ones. Of course, even healthy desserts need to be eaten with
prudence and discretion.

Sweet cravings are natural, and with patience you can
learn to satisfy yours in ways that increase your health
and good looks. Get creative and choose sweet-tasting
foods that are pleasing to your taste buds and beneficial to
your body. Unsweetened apple sauce, a piece of fruit, a
glass of fresh carrot juice, and other natural sources of the
sweet taste will leave you feeling content and cheerfully
energized.

White flour, like white sugar, has had most of its nutritional components stripped away from it and is thus a
partial rather than a complete food. When we eat things
made with white flour, our bodies crave more white flour
in a vain attempt at satisfaction. Cakes, cookies, pies, and
other baked goods that contain both white flour and white
sugar represent a powerfully addictive combination since
they stimulate our appetites two-fold.

In addition to avoiding these sweetened baked goods,
reduce your consumption of white bread, pasta, and other
products made from white flour. Try using whole-grain
bread, which is much more satisfying than white bread, or
better yet, get in the habit of eating the whole grains them-

selves, such as millet, oats, brown rice, barley, etc. Remember that flour plus water equals paste (the literal meaning of *pasta,* after all).

Products made with flour, such as bread and pasta, or other starchy foods, such as potatoes, are great for sticking to your ribs and can be a wonderful source of stamina if you are a runner or engage in other demanding physical activity. For most of us sedentary types, however, the staying power of these foods results only in excess weight.

I love pasta, and I ate it every night of my life until the age of 21, as my ancestors in Italy had no doubt done since the time of Marco Polo. They thrived on it, since they were busy ploughing fields, chopping wood, hauling water, and carrying out all the other activities necessary for survival in an agricultural lifestyle. I, on the other hand, never did anything more active than take a five-minute walk to get to the subway. No wonder my body could not burn off the pasta!

For most of us, modern life means a much less physically active life than that of our ancestors, and our diet needs to be lightened accordingly. Those of us who are overweight need to reduce our intake of carbohydrates. We should avoid starchy products such as bread, pasta, cake, and doughnuts, and we should consume even healthy carbohydrates, such as the whole grains, with moderation.

3. *Avoid very salty foods.* Most people are aware of the negative impact excess salt can have on one's blood pressure, but few people have thought about the effect of excess salt on appetite. I have noticed that excessively salty foods tend to give people cravings for sweets afterwards. If you are accustomed to sprinkling salt on your food, try reducing the amount, and eventually remove the salt shaker from your table entirely.

Although food may taste bland to you in the beginning, once your palate is unclogged from excess salt you will be amazed at how delicious everything becomes. Flavors will seem much stronger than before. Your appetite in general, as well as your appetite for sweets, will become more moderate. Your body craves a variety of tastes, and if you overwhelm it with one taste, such as salt, it is unsatisfied and eternally hungry.

4. *Avoid very fatty foods.* Such foods as pork chops, bacon, cream sauces, mayonnaise, etc., may have been fine for those generations who did heavy physical labor, but most modern, sedentary people cannot metabolize them properly. Like the starches, fatty foods will block and destroy your energy flow if you do not follow a lifestyle of intense physical activity.

5. *Broil, bake, or stir-fry rather than fry.* Fried foods place too much stress on your stomach, liver, and gall bladder, once again disturbing the smooth flow of energy necessary for good metabolism

6. *Avoid microwaved foods.* Microwave ovens are time-saving conveniences, but the fact is that no one knows the long-term effects of eating foods prepared by microwave. I remember that in the 1970s the U.S. government complained that the Soviets were directing microwaves at the U.S. Embassy in Moscow as part of a harassment campaign. The U.S. government claimed that exposure to microwaves was having a deleterious effect on the health of embassy staffers, especially pregnant women.

If the government's claim was true, then it is hard to believe that consistent ingestion of microwaved food can be harmless. In any case, it will be decades before we can fully gauge the impact of microwaved foods on our bodies. It makes sense to avoid a method of food preparation whose long-term consequences are unknown.

7. *Drink plenty of spring water.* Let water be your main beverage. You need pure water, and plenty of it, for high-quality life force. For the sake of your nerves, heart, and

kidneys, reduce your consumption of caffeine and start to think of coffee and tea as beverages you consume occasionally rather than as something you have to have several times a day. Switch to herbal teas and herbal coffee substitutes, or develop the habit of having water when you would ordinarily have coffee or tea.

Soft drinks that contain caffeine should be avoided too, especially since they also contain sugar and/or chemical additives. Alcohol consumption should be kept within safe limits by everyone, and if you are overweight, it is best to avoid alcohol entirely. If alcoholism is a problem for you, please see a good acupuncturist for help and visit a local Alcoholics Anonymous meeting.

8. *Eat lots of vegetables and salads.* Start thinking of vegetables as your main food, even if you are not a vegetarian; let your meat, fish, or whatever you think of as the main food of the meal complement your vegetables, instead of the other way around.

I grew up in a vegetably deprived household; although we had vast quantities of every other kind of food, we seldom had fresh vegetables except for eggplant, lettuce, tomatoes, and cucumbers. Our other vegetables were usually canned or frozen, which was typical of the 1950s when enthusiasm for labor-saving foods was high and nutrition consciousness was generally low.

Now, fortunately, people are more aware of the tremendous vitality and strength that we gain from vegetables, and the variety of vegetables available to us is increasing all the time. Here is just a partial list of the vegetable bounty we can choose from:

Acorn squash, alfalfa sprouts, asparagus, beets, broccoli, broccoli rabe, brussels sprouts, cabbage, carrots, cauliflower, cucumbers, celery, collard greens, corn, daikon radish, dandelion greens, endive, escarole, fennel, green beans, green peppers, kale, lettuce of all kinds, mustard greens, onions, parsnips, radishes, snowpea pods, spinach, sweet potatoes, Swiss chard, turnips, water chestnuts, and watercress.

What abundance!

Make a point of eating root vegetables and leafy vegetables every day. I believe that vegetables are our natural food since they are so brimful of vitamins. Many of us are uninterested in vegetables because our palates have been so ruined by sugar and salt that we cannot discern the delicious taste of vegetables. Once your palate is clear, your attitude towards vegetables will change, and after you increase your intake of vegetables, you will have so much more energy that your appreciation of these wonderful foods will skyrocket.

One of my favorite ways to boost energy is to make a vegetable stew by steaming a variety of colorful vegetables in water mixed with a little olive oil. Try it some time, and feel the charge of life force running through you!

9. *Drink lots of fresh vegetable juices.* Consider investing in a juicer if you do not have a juice bar in your neighborhood. Including fresh juices such as carrot juice, combinations of green vegetables, etc., in your daily diet can have a really dramatic effect on your weight and health.

For a long time I resisted drinking these juices because they seemed like too much trouble to obtain and because the benefits attributed to them sounded exaggerated to me. Was I wrong! The changes in my energy level and figure after just a short time of juicing were really remarkable. I recommend juicing to everyone now.

I am offering these guidelines for food selection for your consideration, and I realize that adopting them may seem like too big a change from your current foodstyle to be comfortable. You do not have to adopt them all at once, and you do not have to adopt them at all if you do not want to. If you do adopt them, I advise you to go slowly, eliminating foods that are troublesome for you one at a time rather than attempting a complete change all at once.

To the extent that you do adopt these guidelines you will be pleased at how much more balanced, strong, and full of energy you feel. Even a small change in the direction of selecting purer food will have beneficial results. As you reap these benefits, your reverence for food will grow and will contribute to your overall appreciation of the physical world and your love for your physical body.

By committing yourself to selecting foods with high-quality life force, you will moreover lift yourself out of a preoccupation with body problems and into a more helpful orientation towards fitness and cooperation with nature. You will be signaling your willingness to support the Divine Intent of increased life, harmony, and perfection on earth.

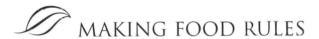 MAKING FOOD RULES

Even if you do not wish to change your current manner of food selection as I have suggested above, something in your current foodstyle will have to change if you wish to lose weight. As I have mentioned before, doing the work outlined in the previous chapters will naturally prepare and incline you towards a more healthful and balanced way of eating. In addition, there are other processes and techniques that you can consciously use to support a beneficial change in your eating habits.

Taking inventory of your current foodstyle is one of these processes. For two weeks, keep a written record of everything that you eat or drink. Many of us eat and drink so unconsciously that we are not really aware of what we are consuming or of how much we are consuming. A written record can be very helpful in objectively appraising your food intake.

YOUR WRITTEN RECORD

When you have compiled your written record, read it through to see the kinds of foods and beverages that dominate your diet. Do you eat lots of creamy foods, sweet foods, starchy foods, fatty foods, or spicy foods? Do you drink lots of soft drinks, caffeine drinks, or alcoholic beverages? Which particular foods keep recurring in your diet? Most of us compulsive eaters have a few foods or types of foods that we are highly fixated on and eat much too frequently.

Sometimes the foods we eat most often are foods which have an immediately noticeable harmful effect on us. For example, we may constantly eat hot dogs, even though they make our veins swell up, or bread, although it makes our bellies distended, or Chinese food prepared with monosodium glutamate, although it gives us headaches.

As part of the addictive/allergic cycle, the negative reactions that our bodies have to these foods produce frequent cravings for the food in question. A varied diet tends to be a light and healthier one, but most of us tend to confine ourselves to the very foods that have had the most harmful impact on our weight and health. Just seeing in written form how repetitive our food intake is can often have a salutary effect.

In addition to foods that we eat too often, there are foods that we cannot stop eating once we start. Everyone has these "trigger" foods that set off wild eating until all trace of the food in question is consumed. What are your "trigger" foods? Jot down as many as you can think of.

Once you are aware of the foods that you eat too frequently, and the foods that are "trigger" foods for you, ask yourself which of these foods it would be most beneficial to eliminate from or decrease in your diet. While we may need some re-education in nutrition to know what to eat, I believe that *if we are honest with ourselves, we all know exactly which foods we as individuals need to avoid.*

After we recognize the foods that we need to cut down on, it can be helpful to make rules to govern our access to these foods. Rules protect and strengthen our resolve to eat wisely. When we make rules about what we'll eat or won't eat, or the circumstances under which we'll eat certain foods, we are establishing useful controls on our interaction with these foods. Rules can give us a sense of relief as well as a feeling of control; it is easier to set rules for eating and follow them than to have to make a decision about whether or not to eat something problematic every time we go to eat.

For example, if you want to cut down on desserts, it is easier to have a rule that says *"I eat dessert only on Sunday"* than to have to face a decision every day about whether or not to eat dessert. If you want to reduce your starch intake, it can help to make the rule *"I always ask for two vegetables with my entree rather than a vegetable and a potato when I eat in restaurants." "I always ask the waiter to take away the bread basket"* is another helpful rule for resisting starch.

MY OWN BEST RULE

The rule that has worked best for me is *"If I can't stop eating it, I don't let it in the house."* Having worked with the principles in this book for so long, my relationship with food is usually tranquil and nonaddictive. There are still a few foods, however, that can trigger me into mindless, compulsive eating if they are around. Since I can't stop eating desserts or chocolates if I begin, I don't allow any sweets in my apartment. I can remember all too vividly the days when I would decide to "Just even off the edge of the cake" and end up eating the entire cake in a matter of seconds!

Mayonnaise is another food that I never keep in the house, because if I used one teaspoonful I would then have to finish the whole jar at a single sitting. It is best to keep such trigger foods out of sight and safely out of mind. You cannot eat what you do not see. If someone you live with can't get used to not having these foods available, then put them all on one shelf in the refrigerator or closet and make a rule that you only eat foods from the other shelves.

SHOPPING RULES

Shopping rules are also necessary. You can make rules about which types of food you will buy and which you will no longer let into your shopping cart, car, and home. To make things easier on yourself, you can also make rules about which aisles in the supermarket you will shop from and which you will avoid. There are other ways as well in which your shopping habits can be changed to support your weight loss effort.

You can buy smaller portions, and you can choose individualized servings rather than larger packages so that you will be more conscious of the amount of calories you are taking in and less tempted to overindulge. You can get out of the habit of really stocking up on food when you shop.

Europeans, who are generally much more normal-weight than North Americans, shop much more frequently than we do and keep far less food in the house. They also cook in smaller quantities, so that left-overs are not created. This seems to be a much healthier pattern, ensuring fresher food and less chance of eating something simply because it is around.

"TRIGGER" FOODS

Trigger foods should be avoided outside the home as well as inside. For example, if pizza is a trigger food for you, make a rule that you do not go into pizza parlors. If your family or friends suggest going to a place where you'll have to see trigger foods, explain that you need to avoid such places for the time being, and suggest an alternative plan.

In my experience, people are usually willing to be flexible and supportive if you give them a chance. If they aren't, realize that they are consciously or unconsciously playing the role of saboteurs. Do not allow yourself to be sabotaged, not even by the most unwitting of saboteurs! A helpful rule for such situations would be *"I only go to places where it's easy for me to eat wisely."*

In time, you will be able to eat anywhere wisely. You will be so pleased with being a more normal weight that you will enthusiastically choose those items on the menu that support your healthier, trimmer body. While you are in transition to healthier eating, however, let rules about where you will eat support your intent and strengthen your determination.

TIMING

Another rule that I have derived great benefit from is *"I never eat after 6:30 at night, except perhaps for a piece of fruit."* If you are overweight, it is a sign that your metabolism and your assimilation are impaired. Whether your excess weight has caused this impairment or whether the impairment has caused your excess weight is irrelevant, since in a cycle of this nature one can intervene at any point in the cycle in order to create change.

The easiest method of intervention is cooperation with the natural rhythm of your metabolism, which is at its highest in the middle of the day and becomes lower in the evening. When you eat your evening meal later than 6:00 or 6:30, it is harder for your body to burn off excess calories. This metabolic difficulty is compounded if you are sedentary for the evening.

If possible, eat your evening meal early, and make it a light meal. If you feel hungry later, snack on fruit, carrot sticks, or some other light treat. Let your midday meal be your main meal whenever you can, to take advantage of your body's metabolic rhythm.

Another way to work in harmony with your body's natural tendencies is to end the practice of eating fruit as part of a meal. Fruit, especially seasonal fruits appropriate to your own climate, can be very beneficial to the body, but its good effects can be interfered with if it is consumed as part of a meal. This is because fruit is digested not in the stomach like other foods but in the intestine. When you eat fruit combined with other foods, your body is under the stress of having to provide digestive processes in two places at once rather than concentrating on the stomach.

A food rule that I have benefited from is "*I eat fruit separately from other foods.*" If you're used to having fruit as part of a meal, try eating it between meals instead and see if you don't feel better and lighter just by this small alteration of your pattern.

The timing of our eating can be as important as the nature of our food. In addition to following the general pattern of our physiology, which puts our digestive and metabolic capacities at their height in the afternoon, we should be attentive to any individual quirks of timing that should be followed in adjusting our eating patterns. For example, you as an individual may tend to gain weight if you eat a certain food at one time of the day, but not gain weight if you eat it at another.

You can take advantage of this personal tendency. Start noticing whether different foods affect you differently at different times of day. In my own case, I have noticed that if I eat something sweet in the morning, I tend to crave and eat sweets all day, whereas eating something sweet later in the day tends to satisfy my sweet tooth rather than stimulate it further. You may want to experiment to see if this is also true for you. It can be very liberating to realize that something previously problematic for you will not affect your weight if you alter the timing of its consumption.

EXPERIMENTING

Experimenting with our individual reactions is important if we wish to maximize change. Breakfast is a good meal to experiment with. Try altering the content of your breakfast and see how this affects your food intake for the rest of the day. If you eat a big breakfast, are you less hungry the rest of the day, or more hungry? It can vary from person to person. If you eat a light breakfast, does your day differ if the breakfast consists of cereal as opposed to a piece of fruit? Is the weather a factor? How do you feel when you eat shortly after waking up as opposed to waiting an hour? Experiment, and then make appropriate food rules based on your findings.

In my own case, it takes me a long time to feel fully awake, so my metabolism isn't very awake either for some time. If I eat even a tiny breakfast soon after waking, my metabolism tends to conk out for the rest of the day. I do much better by waiting. The late Dr. Paul Bragg, one of the pioneers of the health food movement in this country, was famous for saying that a person had to "earn" their breakfast by walking or performing some other exercise to wake up the metabolism. I don't know if this is true for everyone, but it has been helpful advice for me, and I have made a rule to postpone breakfast until I feel awake and hungry.

IS IT REALLY HUNGER?

Hunger is generally a good indication that our body is ready to eat and metabolize. However, many of us, even if we are very obese, do not know how to determine if we are hungry or not. Our hunger for food frequently has nothing to do with physical need and arises rather from a compulsive desire for particular tastes and food textures. This compulsive desire both results from and fulfills our philosophy, our psychology, and our body image.

In my experience, the hallmark of compulsive eating, as opposed to real hunger, is the sense of nervousness that accompanies it. A good rule is not to eat until you are hungry, and a good way of knowing whether you are hungry or not is to ask yourself, *"Am I hungry or am I nervous?"* If you are nervous, find other ways of alleviating your anxiety rather than eating. Do some quick exercises, take a quick walk, or otherwise divert your attention away from food. We will discuss more ways of dealing with nervous hunger below.

Think seriously about the food rules you would like to adopt, and then write them out in a list. You can add to the list as your eating patterns and the way you would like to change them become more obvious. Remind yourself that you are making these rules out of love for your body, and that you can always reevaluate and change the rules as circumstances evolve. Read your list frequently, and allow your rules to guide and support you by governing your decisions about what and when to eat.

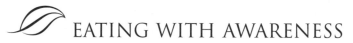 ## EATING WITH AWARENESS

Besides what and when we eat, *how* we eat is also important. We should always eat with conscious awareness of our food, and in ways that can maximize its benefits to us. Many times we wolf down our food without even stopping to taste it, let alone notice anything else about it. Eating in this unconscious way often makes us feel as though we haven't eaten at all. We feel dissatisfied and hungry even if our stomachs are full.

When we eat with awareness, consciously noticing and appreciating our food, we truly experience the act of eating. Our body knows that we have eaten and feels satisfied having consumed a reasonable amount of food, with no need for extra or exaggerated portions. Eating with awareness is an integral part of approaching food with reverence and leads to a new relationship with food, in which our dominant emotion is a sense of satisfaction rather than deprivation.

In order to be truly aware of your food, fully concentrate your attention on it when you sit down to eat. Never listen to the radio, watch TV, or read while eating; eating is a sacred act that deserves your full attention. Energy follows attention, and if your attention is divided between eating and doing something else, you will have inadequate energy for digestion and assimilation.

Always sit down to eat rather than eating while standing or walking. Use dishes and utensils that are a pleasure to look at, and arrange the food on the table and on your plate with care. If you are trying to reduce the size of your portions, *use a plate that is smaller than the size you are accustomed to,* so that your eye will be satisfied seeing a full plate. Notice everything you can about your food before you start eating. What does it look like and smell like? What do you notice about its texture? Appreciate its color, savor its smell, and feel its texture with your fork. Also observe the color and shape of your dishes and eating utensils in detail. Be very present to your food and to these helpful objects.

GIVING THANKS

After you have observed all that you can, give thanks to the Source for the gift of life force that the food contains. Praying over your food before eating is a good way not only to link with Higher Power and align yourself with the life force in the food, but also to increase your appreciation of the physical world. Love for the physical world intensifies when we are conscious of the way the physical universe sustains our life force.

Taking time to notice our food and pray over it is also a helpful means of ending our deep-rooted pattern of instant gratification. Our ability to eat with conscious control rather than automatically can be greatly strengthened through the habit of postponing our eating, even if just for the minute it takes to observe and pray over our food. Once you have gotten used to pausing before eating, you will find it easier to exercise your will and postpone gratification for longer periods. You will no longer be under the compulsive imperative to eat at the immediate sight or thought of food.

INSTRUCTING YOUR FOOD

Before I eat, in addition to observing my food and giving thanks to God for its life force, I also like to address the food directly and instruct it to be of maximum benefit to me. For instance, before a meal I usually pray *"Thank you, my Source, for the life force this food is giving me. Food, I thank you for building my body, and I instruct you to make me trim, attractive, and completely healthy."*

It may sound strange to think of giving instructions to your food, but I have found that doing so creates in me a sense of partnership with food that frees me from emotional dependency on it. I recommend that you add this final step before eating, once you have gotten used to noticing everything about your food in detail and giving thanks.

While eating, pay attention to the taste of the food, so that you will feel satisfied after eating. You must eat slowly enough and chew well enough so that you really experience the taste. Chewing is important not only for the taste experience and the feeling of satisfaction that thorough tasting provides, but also for proper digestion. Be sure to chew each mouthful of food thoroughly, until it is almost liquid. Good digestion is essential to achieve a normal weight, and digestion begins in the mouth and is aided by sustained and proper chewing.

THE IMPORTANCE OF DIGESTION

I was unaware of the importance of digestion in weight loss until I met a doctor of traditional Chinese medicine many years ago who told me that traditional Chinese medicine views obesity and excess weight as problems resulting primarily from impaired digestion. The traditional Chinese medical treatment for persons wishing to lose weight focuses on improving the digestion through acupuncture and herbs. The idea behind this treatment is that if you are not digesting properly, you cannot assimilate needed nutrients from your food, and your lack of nutrition makes you constantly hungry and inclined to overeat. Poor digestion and assimilation moreover lead to poor metabolism as well as unbridled hunger.

If one accepts this traditional theory, then it follows that everyone who is overweight is to some extent malnourished. Malnutrition may be a contributing factor in the increased health difficulties that overweight people seem to experience as opposed to people who are normal weight. Many overweight people tend to have problems with thinning hair and weak nails, two classic signs of malnutrition. Even if we do not have these overt symptoms, however, it makes sense to me that we must be malnourished if we are overweight; we couldn't want to eat so inordinately if we were assimilating nutrients properly. The more you think about this theory, the more it will make sense to you, and you will be willing to chew each mouthful of food as many times as possible in order to improve your digestive capacity and your assimilation.

HAPPY TALK, HAPPY THOUGHTS

When we are eating with other people, we should make sure that the conversation is pleasant. Mealtimes are not the time for arguments, criticism, or the discussion of upsetting topics. For the sake of our digestion, we need to eat in a calm and orderly environment. A friend once told me that in China it was traditionally considered unhealthful to discuss any subject at the dinner table except the food itself!

I have no idea whether this is true, but it certainly is a good idea to limit mealtime conversation to topics that are enjoyable and to avoid any subjects that might give rise to conflict or distress. To eat when angry or experiencing other negative emotions impairs the body's ability to break down food and assimilate nutrients. As you eat, think thoughts of gratitude if the food tastes delicious. If you are alone, you might even say, *"Thank you! This is great!"* out loud. As overweight people, we have been using eating as a means of expressing our unhappiness at the fact of our physical incarnation. When we start to give thanks for the deliciousness of our food, however, eating becomes a means of experiencing God's love for us.

A very wise teacher of mine used to constantly remind us that God usually communicates with us through other people and things rather than in a blaze of direct revelation. Every good thing that comes to us comes from God and is a manifestation of God in our life. When we are aware of food as a gift from our Source, eating delicious food makes us feel loved by God and well provided for.

As we feel gratitude, our love for our Source increases, and we become wrapped in a sense of joy and well-being as each meal becomes an opportunity for us to feel loved and to love back. As our inner peace emerges, it becomes easy for our outer weight to normalize. By expressing gratitude for delicious food, you are transforming the act of eating into an activity that sanctifies you and strengthens your sense of union with the Divine. You are coming to recognize food as an instrument of increased health, attractiveness, and spirituality rather than an instrument of punishment and negative expression.

WHEN ENOUGH IS ENOUGH

Once you learn to eat in this more aware way, it becomes easier to stop eating at the proper time, which is the time when your stomach is comfortably full but not overfull. Many of us eat uncontrollably to the max, so that after a meal we feel totally stuffed and uncomfortable. If your stomach is consistently filled beyond its normal capacity, you are not only taking in too many calories to utilize, but you are also directly impairing your ability to digest and metabolize as a result of this overload. In addition, the stretching of your stomach that occurs from overeating will stimulate increased appetite.

When I was growing up, my father gave me good advice that he had gotten from my grandfather about stopping after an appropriate amount of food. Quoting his own father, my Dad would say "You should get up from the table when you still feel a little bit hungry." I used to feel rebellious at this suggestion, but I realize now that my father didn't really mean "hungry" but rather "with enough room in your stomach so that you don't feel stuffed."

My Dad, significantly, is the only member of my immediate family who has always kept a normal weight, even though he is a hearty eater. God bless my father! It was excellent advice, and I only wish that I had heeded it earlier. Stopping at a point of satisfaction rather than at a point of excess is crucial not only for keeping caloric intake within a normal range but also for developing efficient digestion, assimilation, and metabolism.

AFTER EATING: WHAT?

After you finish eating, it is a good idea to sit peacefully for at least twenty minutes. You can converse, but try not to perform any physical activity during this time, so that your body will not have to meet any demands other than putting your digestive system to work. After 20–30 minutes, go for a walk if you can, in order to help burn off calories. An evening walk after you are through eating for the day can be especially helpful. Since metabolism is generally low during the evening, sedentary habits after our evening meal will exacerbate any tendency we have to put on weight and should be exchanged for physical activity as much as possible.

✍ RAISING METABOLISM

Earlier in this chapter I stressed the importance of following the innate timetable that puts our powers of digestion and metabolism at their natural peak in the afternoon. We can also work to improve our metabolism in general so that we can burn up calories more easily and efficiently.

Many of us who are overweight think that we are stuck with a slow metabolism and that there is nothing we can do about it. We regard with intense envy those energetic friends of ours who can devour vast amounts of food and still have normal-weight, attractive figures or physiques. In keeping with our earlier discussion of dealing with envy, it's important to mentally commend such friends for being masters of metabolism, and to affirm that we want the same mastery and are achieving it with the help of Higher Power.

For this affirmation to work, we must believe that it is possible for our metabolism to change. Too often we resist the idea that our metabolism can change, either from pessimistic disbelief that our physiology could ever change for the better, or because the possibility of improved metabolism seems threatening to our established self-image as an overweight person.

VISUALIZATION TO IMPROVE METABOLISM

We need to remind ourselves frequently that change is possible in this physiological area as well as in other areas of our life. We can also take advantage of the following visualization to safely and effectively improve metabolism:

Sit comfortably, close your eyes, and completely relax. Take three deep breaths with long exhalations, so that you feel even more relaxed. With your eyes still closed, raise your eyes slightly and visualize a beautiful forest that is your own special, private place.

Find a clearing in the forest and notice all the details of the clearing: what it looks like, what sounds you hear there, and what you feel under your feet. Realize that anything that happens in this forest and in this clearing is completely safe and to your benefit. Enjoy looking around the clearing for a minute, all the time feeling more relaxed and secure.

Next let your attention be drawn to a small cottage, located in the clearing, which until now was obscured from your view. The cottage looks very charming; notice the door, the window, the roof, and any other details. Enter the front door and find yourself in the main room of the cottage. Observe the furnishings or other objects that are inside.

Let your attention be drawn to a door leading from the main room into a smaller room somewhat bigger than a good-sized closet. On this door is a sign that says: "Metabolism Control Station." Enter the control station room and see that it is a small engine room full of valves, gears, and machinery in motion. Notice a certain lever (like the lever in a voting booth) that can be moved to three different settings, "Too low, " "Perfect metabolism," and "Too high." Realize that the lever is currently stuck in the "Too low" position. Go to the lever and turn it to the "Perfect metabolism" setting. Know that your metabolism is changing now for the better, and that it is safe and good for you to have a metabolism that is just right. When you are ready, slowly open your eyes and return to normal consciousness. Say out loud *"Thank you for my new, healthy, perfect metabolism."*

Perform this visualization three times a week until your weight loss is well under way, or until you spontaneously see the lever set at the *"Perfect metabolism"* setting in your visualization. There is no need to be held back by a sluggish metabolism; you can change your metabolism by improving your digestive powers through proper chewing, moderate intake, and other means suggested above, and by utilizing the simple but powerful help of visualization.

INCREASING RECEPTIVITY

Inefficient digestion and sluggish metabolism may sometimes indicate a general lack of receptivity on our part. Receptivity does not mean passivity, nor does it mean blind acquisitiveness. Receptivity means our willingness to accept all that nourishes our life and development. When we are resistant to our good rather than receptive to it, our body can express our lack of receptivity by not receiving our food properly, i.e., not digesting and assimilating it. Since we are not receiving the benefits of our food, we are compulsively drawn to take in even more food in a futile and increasingly harmful effort to meet our body's nutritional demands. Thus we take in excessively, but we fail to receive.

Receptivity is the quality connected with the earth element in the traditional categorization of water, air, fire, and earth as the four basic elements from which all things in the physical world derive. The concept of the four elements comes to us from the ancient Greeks, although it existed in even earlier times, and has great symbolic significance. When the elements are understood symbolically, Water represents emotion, Air represents thought, Fire represents activity, and Earth, as I have mentioned, receptivity. For our lives to work well, we need to have the proper balance of heart and mind, and of activity and receptivity. If any of the elements is disordered and is playing too great, too small, or too distorted a role in our lives, it must be adjusted to its proper level and focus.

When we are seriously overweight, we generally have let our level of activity (Fire) fall too low, and our level of emotion (Water) go too high. Our thinking (Air) has become full of negativity and unconducive to our well-being; our receptivity (Earth) at its deepest level is shut down. Increasing receptivity is an important step in bringing ourselves out of the state of excess weight.

ARE YOUR ELEMENTS INTEGRATED?

If asked, most of us would insist that we *are* receptive to our good. While this may be our conscious position, our subconscious mind may take a different stance. To gauge realistically whether or not you are receptive to your good, you can consider whether the Earth element as a whole is successfully integrated into your life.

Each of the four elements "governs" a variety of areas that are correlatives of its main quality. The Earth element governs, as correlatives of its main quality of receptivity, the areas of food, money, pleasure (including, but not limited to, sexual pleasure), creative growth, support, and security. If you have difficulties in more than one of these Earth areas, receptivity in general may be a problem for you.

Being overweight of course indicates difficulties with food, but what about your relationship to the other Earth correlatives? Do you *lack* pleasure in your life, or—at the other extreme—are you *addicted* to your pleasures? Do you chronically lack money, or do you devote yourself to moneymaking so completely that it dominates your life?

Do you lack the opportunity for creative expression in your life, or is your creative energy so diffuse that none of your many projects has a firm enough foundation for success? Do you lack support from family or friends, or are you excessively dependent on the support of others?

Do you feel insecure in your job, relationship, or living situation, or are you so firmly entrenched in the status quo that change seems unthinkable?

All of these conditions of scarcity or excess are symptoms of improper integration of the Earth element and reflect an underlying difficulty with receptivity. *Lack and addiction both come from the same root, which is nonreceptivity to our good.* In the one case, we shut out the things we need; in the other, we let them in, but in a distorted form that can never bring us satisfaction.

VISUALIZATION FOR RECEPTIVITY

The following visualization exercise can help improve your receptivity and foster the proper integration of all the aspects of the Earth element in your life:

Close your eyes and take three deep breaths with long exhalations. Relax. Feel the relaxation moving down your body from the top of your head, down through your face, neck, shoulders, upper body and arms, lower body and legs, and all the way down to your feet. Feel very relaxed and secure.

Imagine that you are lying in the dark in the middle of a circular tower. Though it is dark and confining in the tower, you feel comfortable and safe. It suddenly occurs to you that you can be safe even without the tower.

As soon as you think this thought, you notice that the top third of the tower has disappeared, letting in blue sky and light. Then the second third of the tower disappears, so that you are left with a round wall around you that you could easily climb over if you wished.

Now this last third of the tower also disappears. You get up and you realize that you are in the middle of a vast and very beautiful garden. It feels wonderful to be there.

You intuitively realize that the garden is in the shape of an enormous square. You begin to wander through the garden, marveling at its many beautiful trees, bushes, flowers, and streams. All the riches of nature are in this garden. You enjoy all of the garden's colors and fragrances. You may observe subtle patterns of symmetry in this profusion of beautiful sights—or, on the other hand, the garden may have a completely informal, forest-like quality.

In any case, the garden is enchantingly beautiful. You notice many small birds flying through the garden or nesting there, and gentle animals, such as baby deer and bunnies, living in the rich landscape. You make your way to the periphery of the garden and start walking around the square in a clockwise direction. When you complete your walk around the square, you feel open, receptive, and perfectly secure.

In your visualization you lean down and touch the grass, giving thanks to the Earth for its bounty. Then end your visualization, and sit quietly for a few moments with your eyes still closed. When you feel ready, slowly open your eyes and return to normal consciousness.

Performing this visualization from time to time will be very helpful for bringing the Earth element into proper functioning in your life. When the Earth element is functioning properly, your body will be more receptive to nourishment and will process your food more efficiently. You will also find yourself enjoying more appropriate levels of money, pleasure, creativity, security, and support.

The European alchemists considered Spirit or the Divine force as the fifth element, or quintessence, which brings the other four elements into perfect functioning and harmony. A good affirmation to use to bring all the elements of your life into balance is *"All the elements of my life are coming into perfect order now, though the power of the Spirit."*

MIND SNACKS

You will feel increasingly calm and balanced as you progress on the way of healthy eating. Along the way it can be helpful, as I mentioned earlier, to fortify your new relationship with food by keeping on hand an abundant supply of low-calorie snacks that are not a source of compulsive eating for you. Taking advantage of low-calorie snacks is a good way of avoiding the habit of hunger that frequently derails us when attempting to switch from patterns of excess to a healthier way of eating.

Just as our bodies can profit from healthful snacking, so too can our minds. We can consciously feed our minds with healthful thoughts about food, weight, and our appearance; since our minds then affect our bodies, these "snacks" for the mind provide healthful nourishment for the body just as surely as any carrot stick or radish.

BRIEF AFFIRMATIONS FOR SNACKING

In "mind snacking," we use brief affirmations to encourage ourselves on the path of weight loss. Mind snacking should be done in front of a mirror, preferably a full-length one. Talking out loud to ourselves in front of a mirror gives us very direct access to the subconscious mind as well as a conscious sense of communicating with our body. To give yourself a well-deserved mind snack, stand in front of the mirror and repeat the following affirmations while looking deeply into your eyes:

* You're going to reach your perfect weight of ___ lb., and it's safe.

* It's all right for you to downsize.

* It's all right for you to be healthy, happy, and normal-weight.

✳ It's all right for you to be attractive.

✳ You can be attractive at any weight, and in fact, you're attractive right now.

✳ Your Creator wants you to be healthy, happy, and attractive.

✳ You have a great, new positive attitude towards yourself.

✳ You forgive yourself completely and renounce self-punishment.

✳ You are completely forgiven.

✳ You always treat yourself with love and mercy.

✳ Your weight is becoming a source of happiness to you.

✳ Your digestion, assimilation, and elimination are perfect.

✳ You're developing a wonderful metabolism now. You are a natural fat-burner!

✳ Switching to your perfect weight is so easy for you.

✳ Wonderful things are in store for you!

✳ Wonderful weight loss is coming to you now!

✳ The Infinite desires your success.

✳ God is the creator of pleasure and delight, and your life is a pleasure and a joy.

✳ You appreciate the gift of physical incarnation.

✳ You're at peace with yourself now.

✳ You're at peace with the physical world now.

✳ You're at peace with the opposite sex now.

✳ You are a full participant in life!

✱ You really enjoy this physical incarnation.

✱ You really enjoy eating healthy foods.

✱ You love foods that make you fit and healthy.

✱ You always make excellent food choices.

✱ You're committed to reaching your ideal weight, and you can do it!

✱ Switching to a lower weight is so easy for you, and it's completely safe.

✱ You cooperate with God by becoming healthier, more prosperous, and more attractive all the time.

✱ You activate the Divine in every cell of your body now. Every cell in your body is healthy and happy.

✱ You flow with the Higher Will. You are a being of power and might.

✱ Your life is becoming better all the time. You have lots more fun in your life now.

✱ You are a blessing to everyone around you. You are wonderful!

✱ I love you, and I always let you be happy and healthy.

✱ You are my favorite work of art!

Try to "mind snack" at least three times a week. The affirmations that you state out loud to your reflection in the mirror will not only serve as instructions to your body and subconscious mind but will also cheer and encourage you tremendously. Mind snacking will put you in a wonderful mood, since it provides you with the uplifting experience of giving and receiving love simultaneously. Once you begin mind snacking, you will find yourself automatically smiling at yourself and complimenting yourself every time you look in the mirror. You will become so fond of yourself that it will be easy for you to choose foods that help you look and feel your best and avoid those that hold you back.

You can enjoy regularly scheduled mind snacks, and you can also have a mind snack instead of eating when tempted to eat something that should be avoided. When tempted, go to the mirror instead of the refrigerator. Mind snacking is a major way to deal with temptation, a situation which we'll discuss in more detail below.

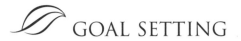 GOAL SETTING

The mirror can be a useful tool when setting goals as well as in mind snacking. Consciously setting goals is important in weight loss, as in any aspect of life, because it focuses the subconscious mind in the direction you desire. When you set goals, you are expressing autonomy over your life rather than accepting all life's vagaries or the inertia of the status quo. Goal-setting helps things happen in your life the way you want them to.

INTERMEDIATE GOALS

We have already discussed the necessity of selecting your perfect weight as part of creating your new self-image. This chosen number is your goal weight. Once you have decided on your goal weight, it's good to set intermediate goals, working down to your goal weight in units of five. If, for example, you now weigh 190 lb. and have a goal weight of 120 lb., your intermediate goal weight would be 185 lb., then 180 lb., etc.

A goal schedule that I found very helpful was to weigh myself every two weeks, aiming each time at my next intermediate goal. (It's important not to weigh yourself too frequently, so that the high numbers of your current weight do not become visually reinforced in your subconscious mind.) More often than not, I did not reach my intermediate goal of a five-pound loss but got at least halfway there. This steady, consistent reduction of two to three pounds every two weeks soon added up to a major weight loss.

To achieve each intermediate goal, it can be very helpful to write down the next number you'd like to reach on slips of paper and put the slips where you'll see them frequently, such as on a mirror, on your desk, near the light switch, etc. Make a point of repeating the desired number to yourself out loud each day while looking in the mirror, and add *"You can do it!"* Whenever you can, imagine yourself getting on the scale and having it register the desired number.

Keep a notebook

You can also keep a written record of your goals and achievements. In a notebook, write down your current weight and the date. Then make a list containing three columns, one column giving dates at two-week intervals, another giving your intermediate goal weights for those dates, and a third in which you will record your actual weight on those dates. Even if you do not achieve each intermediate goal by the proposed date, your list will be a great impetus to progress and an increasing source of satisfaction as you see the numbers come down. You may also find it useful to record your proposed and actual measurements as well as weight.

Your goals do not have to be limited to lists of numbers; you should also set goals based on specific pictures of yourself looking and acting like a thinner person at a certain point in the future, and write out a list of these "picture" goals. The list could include statements such as

"My goal is to fit into my good blue suit again by next spring, when I go to that conference in Denver."
or
"My goal is to wear a size-10 white dress at my graduation in June."
or
"My goal is to lose enough weight by the fall so that I can start jogging around the reservoir."

Read over your list of "picture" goals frequently and keep updating it as goals are fulfilled and new desires occur to you. Goal setting and success go hand in hand. Although setting goals may seem foreign to you in the beginning, eventually you will feel so comfortable with this technique and so convinced of its efficacy that you will want to make a list of goals in all areas of your life for the next year, the next five years, and even longer periods of time.

VISUALIZATION FOR GOAL SETTING

The following brief visualization exercise provides an enjoyable way to support your commitment to your goals and to hasten their achievement:

Sit down in a comfortable position, close your eyes, and relax. Feel the relaxation spreading down your head, through your neck and shoulders, into your chest, down through your stomach and belly area, and into your legs.

With eyes still closed, raise your eyes as though you were looking at a movie screen located several feet in front of you. On the screen see yourself in a large, beautiful, and comfortably crowded banquet hall, where you are approaching the beautifully decorated head table.

As you approach the table, seven celebrities rise to greet you, because you are the guest of honor. The celebrities can be whomever you choose, and they can be from the present time, from history, or mythology. Each celebrity shakes your hand, saying "Congratulations, [your name]! You've done a great job!" and adding other words of encouragement.

Enjoy your interaction with each of these seven celebrities. After they have congratulated you, realize that your whole life is a banquet of wonderful experiences. When you feel ready, slowly return to normal consciousness and open your eyes.

This visualization will help you reach your goals quickly and smoothly. Perform it when you would like to speed up your progress, when you feel the need for encouragement and acknowledgment, or when you would simply like to have fun and be in a great mood.

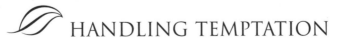 ## HANDLING TEMPTATION

When we are committed to reaching our goals, selecting the right foods and eating them in moderate amounts become second nature to us. Nonetheless, all of us have moments when we are faced with the temptation to eat something that we would be better off avoiding. The following list gives a variety of practical suggestions for dealing with occasions when we experience a strong desire to eat a "trigger" food or some other food that is not helpful:

1. *Remember your goal.* Remembering your goal weight at the time of temptation lets you associate eating with weight, something that most of us who are overweight tend to deny on the emotional level even though we know it intellectually. We have secretly believed that our weight is something that "happened" to us rather than something we ourselves created through eating. When tempted, ask yourself (out loud, if possible), *"Does this food further my goal?"* If the answer is no, tell yourself out loud *"I will not be sidetracked now. My goal is too important. Faster to my goal!"* You can also use the variant question *"Would I rather eat this or be thin?"*

2. *Relieve your nervous anxiety.* Ask yourself *"Am I really hungry, or am I nervous and upset?"* If you are about to eat out of nervous anxiety, try doing something else to alleviate the anxiety. Brief physical exercise or performing routine chores can often alleviate the anxiety enough so that the urge to eat passes.

Another helpful way of dealing with the desire to eat when you are nervous or upset is to articulate your feelings out loud. Articulating your feelings rather than eating will soothe your psyche as well as harmlessly gratifying your oral urges. For example, you can say out loud, "I feel angry and upset because my boss was so vicious at our staff meeting" or "I feel depressed and rejected because I just found out that my ex is remarrying." Identifying the feelings that are causing your nervous hunger and articulating them aloud lets you realize that solace, not food, is really what you want. The relief that comes from describing your feelings out loud can in itself provide enough solace to alleviate nervous hunger.

Remind yourself that food is not solace, and food is not love. If you use food as a substitute for solace and love, your need for solace and love will not be met, and you will feel driven to take in even more food.

For solace and love, turn to other people who care about you, to higher beings such as saints, angels, and your own Soul or Higher Self, and, most importantly, to the Divine. When experiencing nervous anxiety, you can tell yourself, "*All the love and solace I need is available to me now from the right sources.*"

3. *Activate a healthy spirit of competition within yourself.* Tell yourself out loud, "*Other people resist this, and so can I!*" Remember, you only have to resist something a few times for resisting to become easy.

4. *Intervene at the level of your hands.* Unless someone force-feeds you, your hands are what you use to make yourself fat. When facing temptation, break your train of food thoughts by looking down at your hands and saying out loud "*These hands are for helping myself, not for hurting myself.*"

5. *Take several long, deep breaths.* Breathe deeply and hold the breath in your stomach before slowly exhaling it. The life force in the breath will make you feel full enough to comfortably resist temptation.

6. *Breathe purple air.* This technique is especially effective for those times when you are tempted to eat as though there's no tomorrow. Sit down for a minute or two and observe the flow of breath in and out of your nostrils. Then imagine that the air you are breathing in and out is a bluish purple color. Purple is the color traditionally used in spiritual healing to correct addictions and excessive appetites. After a few minutes of breathing purple air, any urge you may have towards inordinate eating will pass and you will once again feel in control.

7. *Have a mind snack.* You can train yourself to head for the mirror and mind-snack when the urge to eat something that is better avoided arises. Even a very quick, abbreviated mind snack will help you refrain from eating foods that set you back.

8. *Say a prayer for help.* A good prayer when you are obsessed with food thoughts or feel like eating compulsively is *"Please let my consciousness be turned in a better direction."*

9. *Remind yourself of food as life-force energy.* Ask yourself *"Is there enough life force in this food to be worth the calories?"* Partial foods, foods with chemical additives, and other types of non-nourishing foods are easy to resist when you think of their low life-force value.

10. *Physically remove yourself from temptation, or temptation from yourself.* Leave the scene if you can, or if the scene is your home, put the temptation back in the refrigerator, or give it to someone else, or put it out in the garbage. Perform some physical action to separate yourself from the food in question, and never be afraid to throw out a food that is troublesome for you.

11. *Consider a substitute.* See if there is something else that you can eat that will satisfy your cravings without negative consequences. For example, if you crave a banana split, you may find that drinking a fruit smoothie made of bananas and other fruit put through a juicer is almost as satisfying. Be creative, and accept your cravings as a challenge to your ingenuity.

12. *Consciously postpone gratification.* As I mentioned earlier, voluntarily postponing the start of a meal, even for the short time it takes to observe and pray over your food, will help break your pattern of instant gratification and give you a new feeling of control over your eating. Postponing gratification when faced with temptation will have even greater results. You will experience liberation from compulsive eating habits and desires, and your will to reach your goal will sharply intensify.

When tempted, tell yourself that you will not eat this food now, but that you can have it in the future if you like; you are not giving it up forever but rather until you reach your final goal weight or an intermediate goal. If the time till you reach your goal seems too far away, tell yourself that you can have it next week, tomorrow, or even an hour from the present, if you feel like it. Your desire may pass during that time, and, if it does not, at least you will be making a conscious choice at the time you eat the food rather than being a slave to impulse.

Many of us who suffer from the need for instant gratification in our eating suffer from it in our other activities as well. Any progress you can make in overcoming the need for instant gratification in other areas of your life will stand you in good stead when food temptations arise. If you *must* turn on the TV the minute you get home from work, try postponing this gratification. If you must run out and buy something the minute you think about it, try postponing your shopping trip instead of shopping compulsively. Your ability to postpone gratification in eating will increase accordingly.

The need for instant gratification comes from deep-rooted insecurity and fears of lack and deprivation. Nowhere is this more apparent than when we are tempted not merely to eat something that we shouldn't but to eat completely uncontrollably. We eat as though there's no tomorrow because at some deep level we fear that tomorrow this food might not be available to us; we gorge ourselves because we really do believe it's now or never. This attitude is often especially strong in us if in our childhood we saw ourselves as being in competition with other family members for food.

A good statement to make out loud when tempted to binge on a certain food wildly or to eat everything in sight is *"I can have this food at any time. This food is always available to me. I choose not to have it for the time being."* You can also imagine your adult self telling your childhood self *"Nobody can take this food away from you. You don't have to eat it all now."*

If you utilize these suggestions, it will become increasingly easy to turn away from harmful food choices when tempted and to opt instead for normal weight and healthy eating. You may find it helpful to use "When Facing Temptation," p. 193. This can be photocopied and carried with you for use anywhere, at any time.

Sometimes as we are learning to overcome our food cravings, we manage to successfully resist temptation, but we feel resentful and deprived in doing so. These negative feelings will generally result in overeating at some later point. To help yourself through these feelings, remind yourself that you are in no way deprived since you already consumed too much at some time in the past, and you are now willingly waiting for balance to re-establish itself. Also remind yourself that your desire to be thinner is more important to you now than the desire for the foods you are giving up. Tell yourself, *"I am gladly giving up rhinestones now for the sake of diamonds later!"*

If you do give in to temptation, be sure to compensate later. Never reproach yourself for eating the wrong foods or too much food; instead, try to compensate by eating more lightly than usual the rest of the day or the next day. If you watch people who are "naturally" trim, you'll find that most of them compensate in this way. If they eat more heavily one day, they'll eat more lightly the next; if they have a big meal at midday, they'll have a light snack in the evening rather than a meal. "Naturally" trim people will eat lunch much later than usual on days that they have had a late breakfast.

We who are overweight, however, tend to eat at least three large meals a day, whether we are hungry or not, and tend to eat at fixed mealtimes even if we are already full at that time. Our natural tendency towards balance has been temporarily lost, and we have become locked into patterns based on habit rather than on the body's innate good sense.

The habit of consistently eating fattening foods or too much food is only a habit and can be changed. Start acting and thinking like someone in balance; strive for moderation and for lighter eating, and if you occasionally overindulge, consciously compensate for the overindulgence.

Compensation does not mean bingeing and purging, or bingeing one day and fasting the next. It also does not mean indefinitely postponing your compensatory light eating to a tomorrow that never comes. We are not talking about any habit of excess or self-deception here, but rather about following the healthy body's natural tendency to judicious choice, balance, and harmony.

GETTING BACK ON TRACK

Sometimes, despite our best intentions, we find ourselves consistently giving in to temptation, or even going off the track of healthy eating completely. Backsliding is especially likely to occur if we eat sweets, since sugar creates such intense cravings for more sugar. Going off the track can happen to anyone, and we must not hate ourselves if it occurs. Rather, we can focus on returning to a balanced way of eating as soon as possible.

If you fall into careless eating habits or notice that excess pounds are creeping up again, remind yourself of why you wanted to lose weight in the first place. Write out a list of your reasons, re-commit to them, and put the list where you will see it frequently. Whatever your specific reasons were, their aim was to increase your freedom, ease, and potential; let this praiseworthy aim re-ignite your desire again. Tell yourself, *"I can do this!"*

Take advantage of motivational tapes, other inspirational books, or other material useful for getting back on track. Remind yourself that of all the things you desire in life, a thinner body is the one most immediately within your realm of possibility, since having it relies only on you.

VISUAL AIDS

Visual aids are often especially useful, and helpful images can vary from person to person. To re-encourage himself, an enterprising teenage boy I knew who had lost a lot of weight used to look at pictures of racing bikes. He loved being light enough to ride a racing bike, and the sight of all those beautiful bikes renewed his determination not to be fat again. When I find myself getting careless, I sometimes put the "Temperance" card from the Tarot deck on my refrigerator as a reminder to avoid excess.

The "Temperance" card in the Visconti-Sforza deck, which was painted in Italy in the early 1500s, shows a woman pouring water from one cup into another, without spilling a drop, while standing on the edge of a precipice. The control and balance depicted in this image remind me to start exercising control again when I find myself close to the precipice of compulsive eating. You can use whatever material you can think of to create an encouraging environment for getting back on track.

ASK YOURSELF

When you find yourself backsliding ask yourself, *"What's going on?" "Why am I doing this?"* and *"What am I saying by regaining weight?"* Carefully review the material given in this book to see where your philosophy, psychology, body image, and attitude towards food need work.

If you reread this book a number of times, it will become automatic for you to start identifying the causes of your excess eating or weight gain as soon as it begins, and you will quickly take steps to liberate yourself from these compulsions. Clarity, purpose, and alignment with the Divine Will to health and happiness will reassert themselves with increasing ease, and balanced eating patterns will naturally be restored. As your familiarity with this book increases, you will become increasingly dedicated to building a carefree, healthy, attractive body as part of your contribution to, and experience of, Paradise on Earth.

5

Experiencing

Paradise Now

B UILDING A CAREFREE BODY can provide us with more Paradise in our lives from the very beginning of our change in eating patterns, since we have the comfort of knowing that we are taking active steps to remove ourselves from the hell or purgatory we have experienced by being overweight. Similarly, any progress we can make in creating Paradise on Earth in other areas of life will also be rewarding from the very beginning. We do not have to wait until the work of creating Paradise is complete to have our lives become suffused with the consciousness of love and union inherent in Paradise. Every contribution we make to our long-term creative work of perfecting the world can immediately reward us with enriched consciousness and increased joy.

Just as we can commit ourselves to reaching our perfect weight as part of our creative mission, we can also commit to other activities and achievements that support the furtherance of Paradise in our personal and societal experience. Such multiple commitments will re-enforce each other and will allow the Higher Self the largest possible scope for implementing its grand design. The more your commitment to creating Paradise on Earth increases, the happier and more integrated into the physical realm you will feel, since you will be doing the work that you came to Earth to do. You will find profound artistic satisfaction and deep enjoyment in seeing your new vision of the world take form.

While expanded commitment can take many directions, I would like to suggest the following primary areas as being particularly conducive to the Paradise state. Some of these areas have been discussed earlier and will be developed further in this chapter, while some are new. These focus areas include Achieving a Sense of Belonging; Expressing Creativity; Learning New Ways of Responding; Assisting in the Feeding of the World; Practicing Meditation Daily; Spreading Divine Light; and Enjoying the Vision of Paradise.

ACHIEVING A SENSE OF BELONGING

To bring more Paradise into our lives, we must feel at home in the world, free of alienation and disaffection. To do this we must achieve a sense of belonging that we as fat people generally have not had. *We become fat because of our fundamental sense of alienation from the physical world, and our experiences as fat people tend to increase our feelings of alienation even more, making us feel alienated from society as well as the physical world.* Chapter One was devoted to ending our alienation from the physical world; here I would like to touch on social alienation.

When we are fat, many of the physical activities, social opportunities, career choices, clothing choices, and other means of expression available to the general population may be outside of our realm of possibility. When whole areas of expression are closed to us, we feel like outsiders. Feelings of inferiority or a lack of self-confidence because of our weight can compound this situation so that we hold ourselves back from attempting things that would otherwise be open to us. Popular culture, with its emphasis on thinness, can also make us feel marginalized and outside of the mainstream of life.

Overweight people frequently encounter prejudice from others, particularly in areas of social acceptance and employment. Discrimination by salespeople can also be a problem. Prejudice is based on fear, and normal-weight people who subconsciously fear fat people do so because our evident lack of control over our eating reminds them of some lack of control in their own lives that they fear.

Eventually, we will all stop reacting to each other with fear and will view each other with hope and compassion instead. Until that time, those of us who have been marginalized by our physical bulk, or own hesitation, or society's prejudice should do all we can to overcome our feelings of alienation and develop a sense of belonging. If we do not feel that we belong to a greater whole, we are as psychologically insecure as if we were dangling alone in space. We must feel part of a larger group or enterprise whose goals we share and whose interests resonate with the interests of our own souls. In other words, we must find a group or endeavor that feels like our spiritual home and actively enjoy the sense of common purpose our membership in this group brings.

FINDING A GROUP

Look for a group that can provide you with a sense of spiritual home. Become committed to finding a group whose activities bring out the best in you and whose sense of purpose is dear to your heart. It may be a group concerned with spiritual pursuits, community service, sports, exercise, other hobbies, or cultural, charitable, or intellectual interests. The key factor is that the group's activities are meaningful to you at a very deep level of your being.

I've known people who have achieved a sense of belonging and found a spiritual home in such diverse environments as an ice skating class, a volunteer ambulance service, and a Revolutionary War discussion club, to name just a few! Their participation in these groups gave them an opportunity for self-expression and a sense of united purpose that brought them out of alienation and into the feeling of meaningful connectedness associated with Paradise.

WHEN IT'S THE WRONG GROUP

If you've already been participating in a group activity and still have a serious weight problem, your group has not alleviated your feelings of social alienation, although it may have provided you with other benefits. Some groups can even increase their members' sense of alienation instead of providing them with a sense of spiritual home; this is particularly the case when a group is fraught with divisiveness or controlled by negative personalities. It's a good idea to withdraw from groups filled with hostile members and from activities that consist of unwanted, burdensome obligations.

Sometimes we become part of a group not out of real interest but because we *think* we should; for example, you might become active in a fund-raising campaign for a charity because you are good at fund-raising and are being pressured to help the group, even though this activity does not bring you joy. To continue with this activity would only lead to increased feelings of alienation in the long run.

Sometimes we become part of a particular group because we know that we can dominate the group and thus have another venue in which to "throw our weight around." In such a case, it can be helpful to take a lesser role and learn to enjoy participation in the group without dominance. If our group is to be a spiritual home, it should bring out the best in us and not re-enforce our old patterns of negative behavior.

TOO MUCH GIVING?

Sometimes our group activities require too much giving from us when what we really need is more receiving. This is especially true of religious workers, social workers, nurses, child-care workers, and others in demanding occupations who are always giving to others. People in these occupations frequently have weight problems because they give so much that there is no time to receive, and nonreceptivity, as noted in the last chapter, results in nonassimilation of nutrients, consequent food cravings, and fat. The group activities these people are drawn to are frequently an extension of their professional roles and do not nurture them in ways they need. If you are in one of the "giving" occupations, look for a group or activity that is not connected with giving but is rather one in which

you have fun and enjoy yourself. Fun is an excellent antidote to burn-out and feelings of alienation.

NETWORKING

In addition to belonging to a meaningful group that gets
together in person, we can also help overcome feelings of
alienation by becoming part of a network of people who
are working for the same purpose even though they seldom or never meet. For example, I belong to the Quartus
Society, a metaphysically oriented group whose founder,
John Randolph Price, originated the World Healing Day
meditation for world peace which millions of people participate in annually on December 31st.

I have never met Mr. Price or any other Quartus members, but I derive tremendous support from receiving the
Quartus newsletter and knowing that through the Quartus
Society I'm connected with people who truly desire a
world of peace, prosperity, and creative self-expression for
all. I encourage you to similarly become part of a nonlocal
organization whose work is meaningful to you. Your sense
of belonging will greatly increase as you realize that at a
deep level you are linked with large numbers of like-
minded people spread throughout a large geographic area
or even throughout the world.

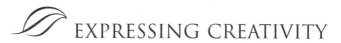 EXPRESSING CREATIVITY

As I've emphasized many times in this book, our Higher
Self is creative by nature and took on physical form for the
enjoyment of creating Paradise on Earth. The more we let
our personal creativity flourish, the more consonant we
are with the nature of our Higher Self. When we are
engaged in creative work, whether it is baking a cake,
painting a picture, setting our company's goals for the
next five years, or figuring out a way to fit a grand piano
through a narrow hallway, we tend to experience the

Paradise qualities of satisfaction and joy. We must express our creativity as much as possible if we are to be happy. No frustration is greater than that of creative frustration; we all need an outlet for creating something of personal, group, or societal value.

To allow our creativity its maximum expression, we should do everything possible to develop our talents and skills. This is one of the greatest priorities of the creative mission for which we came to Earth; when we learn to do something valuable that we could not do before, or when we bring our meaningful accomplishments to an even higher level, we are carrying out the evolutionary directive of our Higher Self.

These achievements result in joy and increased self-esteem since they are gratifying to us at a deep level as fulfilling our mission. Such achievements can also result in a new self-image. In addition to all the suggestions given in Chapter Three, learning to do something new or to do something better is a speedy way to help transcend the old image that keeps us locked in the past.

We all have talents and abilities, even if we have not tapped or developed them yet. Become committed to exploring your as yet undeveloped talents as part of your dedication to creating Paradise on Earth. If you are uncertain as to which direction to go in, start with your childhood interests and aspirations. If you enjoyed writing, drawing, singing, or building things as a child, but never perform these creative activities now, the chances are that you have a natural affinity for these activities that you may have suppressed at some point out of insecurity or fear of failure. Start doing them again for your own pleasure and self-development.

FROM VIEWER TO DOER

The same applies to those activities for which you love to be part of the audience, but which you have never actively participated in yourself. For example, if you love going to the opera or to concerts but have never sung or played an instrument yourself, treat yourself to some voice or music lessons. The chances are that if you enjoy watching an art form, sport, or other activity, you will enjoy doing it yourself, even if in a highly modified form. When I was a teenager, I used to love to watch track meets, and I especially admired Wilma Rudolph, the Olympic champion who had overcome childhood polio to become one of the great female runners of all time. Since I was five feet tall and weighed over 200 lb., there was no way that I could be a runner, although running was one of my secret dreams. Now that I am at a normal weight and could run if I wanted to, I don't do so because I live in New York City and I don't like the idea of running on concrete or in indoor tracks. However, I do fulfill this secret dream of my past in a modified way by being a prodigious walker. I walk three miles a day very rapidly, and I thoroughly enjoy the sensation of speeding along. Walking is not usually thought of as a talent or skill, but it gives me the self-expression and satisfaction of a talent or skill, and I claim it as one of mine.

MODIFIED FORM IS OK

Finding a modified form for certain talents or skills is especially useful when we are too overweight to develop them in the usual way. For example, if you are very heavy and you always wanted to be a ballerina, you can at least learn ballroom dancing or some other type of dancing that is possible for you until you are trim enough to learn ballet for your own enjoyment. Similarly, if you have always wanted to play tennis but have been too heavy to run back and forth, you can at least play ping-pong now, so that your hand/eye coordination will be well developed when you are ready for tennis.

Running in place is a very good skill to develop if you are too overweight for distance running but not too overweight to run at all. If you run in place to the count of 100 every day, your body will start to tone up and your metabolism will receive a nice boost. Start slowly and gradually work your way up to the count of 100. This very quick and simple exercise can have excellent results.

Some of the simplest physical skills, such as skipping and jumping, can often bring us the greatest joy. Most of us have not skipped or jumped since childhood. Try skipping or jumping now, and see how wonderful it makes you feel! I believe that depression could be eliminated in many cases if we took up these simple, joy-producing skills again.

Your Higher Self wants to express its creativity and expertise in all areas of your life. Let this inner longing find an outlet through your talents and skills. There is no limit to the beautiful things that can be created, the successes that can be achieved, or the fun that can be had, and you will never know what you are good at if you do not try. We are constantly able to develop, express, and enjoy ourselves, so that our lives become more reflective of Paradise.

LEARNING NEW WAYS OF RESPONDING

In Paradise all people dwell in harmony. Become committed to having harmonious relationships in your life, including harmonious relationships with mates or lovers, family members, friends, neighbors, bosses or co-workers. In order to have more harmonious relationships, we generally must learn new ways of responding to those aspects of other people's behavior that get on our nerves.

In Chapter Two I mentioned the need to seek peaceful solutions to relationship difficulties so that we don't subconsciously resort to using excess weight as a weapon. Here I would like to stress the same need in all our daily interactions, so that we can experience comfortable encounters rather than constant strife.

If we want to enjoy harmonious living, we must learn harmless and productive ways to react. There are many excellent books and tapes available now that can teach you how to express anger and annoyance constructively and without escalating tensions. Go to your library or bookstore and find the specific advice you need for coping with the difficult people in your life and converting strife to peace.

We are very fortunate in having such a wealth of constructive practical advice available to us. These materials can teach us simple ways of changing criticism into less critical statements that can get our point across more successfully, such as, for example, telling a teenager "I need some quiet time," instead of "You're driving me crazy with that music."

THE "EVOLUTIONARY" RESPONSE

As a general guide for responding to an annoying person or troublesome situation, it is good to ask yourself, *"What is the best thing that I could do or say here for the higher evolution of everyone concerned, myself included?"* If you start thinking about the most "evolutionary" response you can make, your perspective on the situation will grow larger, and new ideas for constructive dialogue or correct action will occur to you. What to say or do and when and how to say or do it will become more evident. You will become more skilled at expressing your feelings without worsening a situation. You will have a better understanding of when a situation can be healed and when the most evolutionary choice would be for you to leave the situation.

Frequently I am not clear about the most evolutionary choice I can make in a situation, and I wonder if what I am about to do or say will really be beneficial or whether it is just a customary, nonproductive response making its appearance in a disguised form. In such cases I try to refine my idea of evolutionary behavior by remembering the concept of *theosis* taught by the early Fathers of the Christian

Church and developed most beautifully in Eastern Orthodoxy. *Theosis* is Greek for "deification" or " becoming God." It refers to the process by which human nature is perfected, sanctified, and made glorious by the indwelling of the Holy Spirit. Since I have a Christian background, theosis is a meaningful concept for me, and it provides a clear standard by which I can recognize an evolutionary choice. I can ask myself *"Will what I am about to do or say promote theosis, or slow it down?"* I usually become clearer about my motivations and the appropriateness of my response if I ask myself this question.

If you have some specific concept of higher evolution that is particularly meaningful to you, you can utilize that concept or definition as a standard for judging whether your choice is evolutionary or not. Become committed to asking yourself whatever questions are appropriate for you to help you choose evolutionary behavior over a nonproductive or even harmful response.

Of course, sometimes no matter how much we would like to make an evolutionary choice, and no matter how many questions we might ask ourselves, we wind up just "losing it,"—losing control and losing our tempers. This is inevitable at times, and it should not discourage us. We are all so used to responding without thinking of the consequences that it may take a long time for us to break away from old patterns and adopt a more helpful perspective. At least we can try to move in this newer, more liberating direction.

COMPASSION IS APPROPRIATE

We can increasingly try to see difficult people as travelers on the evolutionary journey who have temporarily forgotten their destination and taken a detour into difficult behavior to fulfill some emotional need. We can cultivate compassion for these people, for ourselves in having to deal with them, and for ourselves when we are being difficult or uncooperative. At the same time we can equip ourselves with helpful knowledge from the wealth of psychology and self-help materials available to us on the subject of responding productively.

We can take an evolutionary view when responding to our own needs as well as when responding to others' behavior. In Paradise all our needs are met. Become committed to asking other people for what you need. Other people are not mind-readers and cannot know what you need unless you tell them. Make your requests specific. For example, if you feel overwhelmed by your family responsibilities, ask a trusted friend or relative for two hours' worth of child care, elder care, shopping assistance, etc. If you feel overwhelmed at work, ask your supervisors for additional help with specific tasks or in specific heavy periods. Speak up, and believe that your needs can and will be met. This technique may not always be successful, but you will wind up with more help if you ask for it than if you never make your needs known.

WHEN WE NEED ATTENTION

Sometimes we need attention rather than specific help. Instead of unconsciously demanding attention by overeating and gaining weight, or by other negative behavior, we can ask consciously for attention instead. At first this idea may seem strange. I myself was surprised when a friend once called me and said, "Can you invite me to dinner one night this week? I'm calling everybody I know, because I need attention." Her business was failing, and she felt depressed.

Although I was at first taken aback by her request, I was actually very glad that she asked. I didn't want her to equate dinner with attention, so I suggested that instead of making dinner for her, I would treat her to a special exhibition at the Metropolitan Museum. She was pleased with the suggestion, and instead of feasting on food, we feasted on Matisse.

Since then I have been a firm believer in asking for attention when you need it. I have noticed that people who ask for attention tend to recover more quickly from whatever upset feelings they have been experiencing. They do not need to manipulate, seethe in self-pity, fume, or act out; they simply ask, and they usually get what they need.

Asking does not mean badgering or whining; it means a straightforward, finite request. Asking for what you need is frequently the most evolutionary choice you can make when you are feeling upset, neglected, or overwhelmed. It is certainly a better choice than overeating!

Become committed to responding to your own needs by asking for whatever help or attention you require; make it part of the process of creating Paradise, in which your own inner harmony is restored as well as your harmony with others.

ASSISTING IN THE FEEDING OF THE WORLD

While honoring our own needs, we must not forget that much of the world's population has very basic needs that have not been met. Food is a primary need among vast numbers of our world family; hunger and starvation are rampant in so many areas of the world. As people who are fat or overweight, we know what a compelling force hunger can be and what a powerful grip it can have on us.

Our hunger has been so intense, and it has not even been based on physical deprivation; imagine how painful and desperate true hunger must feel! We who have experienced the hunger of compulsive eating are in a unique position to empathize with our brothers and sisters who endure the hunger caused by lack of food.

Since hunger is something we know so much about, relieving the hunger of others is an especially appropriate contribution we can make to establishing Paradise on Earth. When we assist in the feeding of the world, we are manifesting the loving care, sharing, and abundance that are characteristic of Paradise. By participating in hunger relief we can also help free ourselves from domination by food, since feeding those whose lives are imperiled by lack of food will support our reverential attitude towards food and the life force it contains and confers.

ORGANIZATIONS

Become committed to alleviating hunger. Contribute your money, time, food, or other assistance to feeding those who are in need. Every community has soup kitchens, food banks, and other local relief efforts that could use your help. There are also many nonprofit international aid organizations, such as the International Rescue Committee, Catholic Relief Services, etc., which need your financial contributions to perform their heroic work of feeding people who live under dire conditions of famine, war, or natural disaster.

One of my favorite groups to contribute to is the Rodale Institute, located in Emmaus, Pennsylvania. Rodale specializes in teaching small farmers methods of organic agriculture which enrich the soil and so increase crop yield, enhance the environment, and foster local self-sufficiency. Rodale has projects in the U.S., Senegal, Guatemala, and Russia. Your library will have information about other local and international organizations, as well as their addresses. Get involved either in a hands-on way or at a distance, and let relieving hunger be a major part of your commitment to creating Paradise on Earth.

A TALE OF TWO BROTHERS

To encourage you in this work, I would like to retell for you an inspiring Jewish tale from Eastern Europe about fraternal love and sharing that I once heard told by a rabbi in New York:

Once upon a time there were two brothers whose farms were located at some distance from each other. One brother had a devoted wife and lots of children, while the other brother was unlucky in love and never married. At the end of the harvest, each brother started thinking about the other. The brother who had no family said to himself, "My brother has so many more obligations than I do, what with all his kids. I should share my harvest with him, since he needs it more than I do." This childless brother decided to drive his wagon full of grain and vegetables to his brother's field in the middle of the night and secretly leave the food there. Meanwhile, the brother with all the children said to himself, "My brother is all alone, with no wife and children to take care of him if anything should go wrong. I should share my harvest with him, since he needs it more than I do." This brother with all the children decided to drive his wagon full of grain and vegetables to his brother's field in the middle of the night and secretly leave the food there.

Each brother loaded his wagon and set off in the middle of the night. At the midpoint between the farms, they suddenly caught sight of each other by the light of the moon. When each brother saw the other brother's wagon full of food, he instantly perceived what his brother was doing. Filled with love for each other, the brothers embraced each other and praised God.

Isn't this a wonderful story? If we all were like these brothers, how quickly the world would be transformed!

MEDITATING DAILY

To expedite the transformation of ourselves and the world, nothing is more useful than the daily practice of meditation. Meditation can alleviate one's sense of being burdened, as I mentioned in Chapter Two, but it can also do far, far more. Meditation changes us at a very deep level, bringing out our potential for greater wholeness in all our concerns, whether personal or societal.

Meditation relieves stress, dissipates feelings of alienation, promotes health, and activates our innate capacity for organization so that we automatically find ourselves accomplishing far more in any given time period than we would have had we not meditated. The life-changing benefits of meditation cannot be overstated, and the meditators who claim that it offers the answer to all the world's ills are in no way exaggerating.

MANY FORMS, ONE GOAL

There are many different forms of meditation, but all aim at emptying the mind of its usual thoughts so that a deeper level of being is experienced. Hatha yoga, Tai-Chi, Qi Gong, and other motion-based forms of meditation utilize specific movement and breathing patterns to bring about this state of deeper harmony with the universal life-force. Seated forms of meditation utilize breathing, visualization, or the repetition of mantras to bring one to this deeper state in which the peaceful, blissful, ever-renewing level of consciousness is experienced.

Some methods of meditation are more devotionally based than others and have as their goal a transcendental sense of union with the Divine. Contemplation is the term traditionally given to this type of meditation. Some methods focus on greater mental clarity, while others foster greater compassion. There is a form of meditation valuable for every personality type and disposition.

SILVA MIND METHOD/TM®

If you are unfamiliar with seated meditation and would like to learn to do it, the two organizations that I would most recommend are the Silva Mind Method and Transcendental Meditation (TM®). Though these two organizations have very different orientations, the former focusing on immediate, practical applications of accessing a deeper level of mind and the latter emphasizing the shifts in consciousness that arise as a result of meditation practice, they both have been widely active since the 1970s and have extensive experience in introducing beginners to a new level of being. The Silva Method does not use the term meditation but rather talks about entering the "Alpha state" of brainwaves, which is the state experienced in meditation. TM® is based on Indian spirituality, but the meditative technique they teach does not require any particular beliefs. You can check the telephone book in any large city to locate the local Silva Method office or TM® Center near you.

Become committed to meditating every day, once if that is all you can manage, but twice for greater efficacy. You will not only enjoy the Paradise-like experience of a more blissful consciousness, but you will also find yourself on automatic pilot for the more effective creation of Paradise on Earth.

 # SPREADING DIVINE LIGHT

Just as meditation is one of our great unseen instruments for creating Paradise on Earth, Divine Light is another. Mystics from every great spiritual tradition have seen that the physical world is suffused with the radiant, unifying, loving, intelligent light of God. Dante, the great poet of Divine Light, describes this light in the *Paradiso* section of his *Divine Comedy* as "light intellectual, light full of love, love of true good, love full of joy, joy that surpasses every sweetness."

Contemporary physics lends support to this spiritual vision of the omnipresence of Divine Light by positing that light is the underlying basis of all matter. Most of us never think about Divine Light. The term *Divine Light* may be familiar to us from religious or philosophical studies, but it is not a term that we hear very often, and most of us do not consider Divine Light a concept relevant to our daily lives.

Fortunately, the time for widespread ignorance about this great treasure that permeates our world is passing. As our evolution proceeds and we make greater progress in spiritual understanding, we are naturally becoming more conscious of the omnipresence of Divine Light. We are also becoming open to the idea of accessing Divine Light in order to eliminate suffering and bring about Paradise on Earth.

YOU ARE MADE OF LIGHT

You can begin now to accept the idea that Divine Light is within you and all around you. As a good starting-point, you can remind yourself daily that we are made of Light and that the brilliance of this Light becomes more evident when we act with love towards ourselves and others. Divine Light is not just a metaphor: it is really here.

We can "spread" the Light, or more accurately, reveal it, by doing whatever we can to alleviate suffering and promote the healing of the world. In this great work, the Light can be our instrument and our end, as well as being the encouraging sign of the Paradise-potential inherent in the physical plane.

SPIRITUAL HEALING

Nowhere is the Light more readily available to us as an instrument than in the area of spiritual healing. By spiritual healing is meant that healing that comes directly to us from our Source rather than through the valuable intermediaries of medicine, herbs, massage, exercise, or other healing modalities. Many forms of spiritual healing rely on Divine Light.

From the earliest history of Christianity, Christians have invoked the "light of Christ," or the Divine Light incarnated in Jesus, in prayers for healing and protection. Divine Light has also been an important aspect of healing in many Eastern traditions, most notably in meditation on Amida Buddha, the Buddha of light. In recent times a number of newly developed or rediscovered systems of spiritual healing that utilize the flow of Divine Light through the hands have made their way from Asia to the West.

These systems of spiritual healing use various frequencies of Divine Light and often feel quite different from each other, even when they have external similarities. As in all healing methods, one system may be more beneficial for an individual than another, since we are all constituted so differently from each other. Two of these Light-based systems that I am familiar with are Reiki and Johrei.

REIKI/JOHREI

Reiki is an ancient Tibetan system of healing through the hands which was introduced to America from Japan in the 1970s by the late Mrs. Hawayo Takata. Reiki is generally translated (from the Japanese) as "universal life-force energy." In Reiki, the universal energy of Divine Light is transmitted to the recipient through the laying on of hands by a Reiki practitioner.

Johrei means "purification of the spirit." The founder of Johrei was Mr. Mokichi Okada, known to members of the Johrei Fellowship as Meishu-sama, who lived in Japan from 1882 to 1955. In Johrei, a practitioner directs Divine Light through his or her hand towards the recipient in order to purify the recipient's "spiritual body," of which the physical body is a reflection. The giving of Johrei is one of the three main activities of the Johrei Fellowship, which is actively dedicated to the creation of Paradise on Earth. The other two activities are "Nature farming," which is a biodynamic method of organic agriculture, and flower arranging, practiced for the soothing and elevating effect of floral beauty.

I have received and given both Reiki and Johrei, and I greatly recommend these two methods of spiritual healing. Like most spiritual healing methods, their impact is gradual rather than immediate, but nevertheless profound. They relieve stress, promote emotional balance, and facilitate physical improvement. They can be a very valuable adjunct to whatever else you are doing to heal your health and weight.

WHERE TO TURN

If you would like to experience Reiki, your best bet (if you do not have a personal referral) would be to look in any publication where holistic-health practitioners advertise, or to check with your local organic-foods store, where Reiki practitioners often have ads posted. There is no central Reiki organization, although there are different groups or alliances of Reiki practitioners.

For information about the existence of a Johrei center near you, you can contact the national headquarters of the Johrei Fellowship, in Torrance, California. The Fellowship is legally organized as a religion, and some Fellowship practices are those of traditional Japanese religion, but there is no need to join the Fellowship to receive Johrei. Johrei centers are staffed by Fellowship members who gladly give Johrei to anyone who comes in to receive it.

YOU TOO ARE A HEALER

Many other forms of spiritual healing exist, suitable for whatever your spiritual inclination or religious background. I encourage you to learn about spiritual healing so that you can help yourself and others. I believe that we can all be healers; healing is part of our potential as spiritual beings engaged in the creation of Paradise on Earth.

Even if you do not feel drawn towards practicing spiritual healing in a formal way, you can at least develop the habit of "sending" healing light to someone in need of it, by an act of your will. When you think of someone who is ill, agitated, or otherwise distressed, think, *"I am sending you Divine Light to heal and strengthen you."* Imagine the person surrounded by the Light and getting better. You can also do this for distressed areas of the world.

Mystics tell us that Divine Light is responsive to us, and scientists confirm that light is responsive to the observer. Light behaves sometimes as a particle and sometimes as a wave, and which one it is can be influenced by the intent of the observer. Don't let the omnipresent resource of Divine Light go neglected and unutilized. "Wrap" yourself in Divine Light every day, affirming *"I am wrapped in Divine Light for my healing, protection, and perfection."* Enjoy the light as you use it to create Paradise on Earth.

MAINTAINING THE VISION OF PARADISE

Another enjoyable means of creating Paradise on Earth is to consciously hold the vision of Paradise each day. By so doing you are affirming Paradise on Earth as your goal and shifting into the vibration that will eventually cause it to manifest. As you go about your daily routine, imagine what conditions would be like if we were living in a Paradise. For example, if you are riding to work on a train or subway, visualize what conditions would be like if the system were completely comfortable, clean, and safe. Visualize what your fellow-travelers would look like if they were completely happy, healthy, prosperous, friendly, and enthused about where they were going.

If you drive to work, visualize what it would be like if your vehicle were completely nonpolluting and ran on some fuel or power whose production and emissions had no harmful consequences for the Earth or any being on it. Imagine what it would be like if other drivers were always courteous and careful, and accidents were a thing of the past.

Similarly, when you read, see, or hear a disturbing news story, take a minute to imagine what it would be like if the opposite of the crime or other disaster reported had occurred. Think about how you would feel if you were learning wonderful news, such as peace being declared in some war-torn area, or the discovery of a miracle cure for some disease, or some remarkable instance of people helping each other. It is important to strengthen the possibility of such things happening by thinking about them and keeping them in our consciousness as desired goals.

You can even imagine what it would be like if natural disasters no longer occurred but were replaced by amazing, nonharmful displays of the majesty of nature instead, such as massive new forests appearing, or beautiful islands coming to the surface of the ocean! In Paradise, any good thing is possible, so let your creative imagination really indulge itself. I sometimes like to imagine how wonderful it will be when I can eat whatever I want and always be healthy and trim!

You can make it a habit to mentally wish good health and well-being for anyone you see suffering from illness, emotional distress, or any other problem—and imagine how good it will be when we are *all* healed, prosperous, and purposeful. You can also wish good things for the people around you when you are waiting in line at the bank, supermarket, etc. This will not only expedite the creation of Paradise on Earth but will also relieve you of much of the boredom and frustration of waiting.

While you are at it, you can also imagine what it would be like if everyone were helpful and efficient, and there was always plenty of time for everything you wanted to accomplish! Life as we have known it has been full of ups and downs, and while we may not be immune yet from suffering or difficulty, we can at least prevent our mindset from being permanently affected by them by imagining what a different, *perfect* world would be like.

VISUALIZATION OF PARADISE

A favorite visualization of Paradise that I like to perform, especially when I am feeling beaten down or thrown off course by circumstances or my own mood, is one that I have devised based on Dante's complex and magnificent vision of Paradise in the Divine Comedy. If you would like to perform this visualization, read it through many times before beginning, even if you are using a tape. Since this is a long visualization, you might even like to practice it in segments for a period of time before performing the entire visualization.

In this visualization, we will travel as Dante did in his *Paradiso* beyond the earth into 10 spheres of Paradise concentrically surrounding the earth—and beyond the 10 spheres to the highest level of Paradise, the Empyrean. In this visualization we are not concerned with the specific theological, philosophical, and historical content of this masterpiece of late medieval Christendom. Rather, we are concerned with the uplifting power of the structure of Dante's ascent into higher and higher levels of Paradise, and with the richness of certain of his images.

I must mention that in Dante's vision, every soul in Paradise is filled with bliss to his or her own capacity, and while certain blessed souls may dwell in one of the 10 spheres, they are all also dwelling in the Empyrean. To occupy any level of Paradise is to experience the bliss of the highest level. Thus we are rising vertically through what appears to be a hierarchy of experiences, but there is no hierarchy of bliss here, only a universality.

THE MOUNTAINTOP

To begin, close your eyes, take a deep breath, and slowly exhale. Repeat this deep inhalation and slow exhalation twice more. Relax your whole body, feeling the relaxation spread down through your head, neck, shoulders, arms, upper torso, lower torso, legs and feet. Feel completely and deeply relaxed.

With your eyes still closed, visualize yourself at the top of a very high mountain accompanied by a guide whom you trust completely. The guide may be your guardian angel, a saint or other holy person, or any figure you regard as a benevolent, protective presence with a higher level of spiritual understanding than your own.

On top of this mountain at the top of the earth, your guide leads you into the Garden of Eden.

THE GARDEN OF EDEN—BEAUTY

Here, in the original prototype of Paradise on Earth, you see wonderfully beautiful trees, flowers, rivers, and other elements of nature. In this garden, you can enjoy nature in its most beautiful and life-supportive state.

Feel completely welcome here, and feel that you are in harmony with a loving, sustaining Earth. Feel cared-for and provided-for. Then when you feel ready, ask your guide to help you ascend into Paradise.

See yourself ascending with your guide through a rarefied atmosphere into the first level of Paradise, called *The Heaven of the Moon*.

THE HEAVEN OF THE MOON—SERENITY

In the Heaven of the Moon, observe a beautiful, tranquil evening sea, with a moon as white as a pearl shining above it. Allow yourself to be filled with the serenity of this scene. Let this feeling of serenity flow through every part of your body, filling you with calmness, peace and contentment.

After you have enjoyed this feeling of serenity, ascend with your guide to the next level of Paradise, the Heaven of Mercury.

THE HEAVEN OF MERCURY—JUSTICE

As the Heaven of the Moon is associated with serenity, so the Heaven of Mercury is associated with justice, meaning the restoration of all things to rightful balance. In this Heaven, allow an image of justice or restoration to come into your mind. It might be the image of a pair of scales coming into balance, or the image of a judge issuing a wise decree, or the image of a king inviting others to take what they want from his granary, or any other scene that to you symbolizes an increase in equilibrium.

As you regard this image, feel happy that restoration to balance is being made. Then imagine that any imbalance in your life, whether of weight, emotion or life circumstances, is being restored to proper balance.

Feel the happiness and relief of your personal restoration to equilibrium. Enjoy this sensation, and when you are ready, ascend with your guide to the next sphere of Paradise, the Heaven of Venus.

THE HEAVEN OF VENUS—LOVE

The Heaven of Venus is associated with love, both

romantic and familial. In the Heaven of Venus, see someone you love. Let a feeling of love fill your heart as you regard this beloved person. If there is no one whom you love, see instead a symbol of love. You might see a famous pair of lovers joining hands, a Valentine heart, a Madonna and child, or any other image of the romantic or familial love you desire.

Ally yourself with this symbol and affirm that you too will experience love in the future. Feel the love for a future beloved mate or for a child fill your heart. When this loving feeling has made you feel happy and buoyant, ascend with your guide to the next sphere of Paradise, the Heaven of the Sun.

THE HEAVEN OF THE SUN—WISDOM

The Heaven of the Sun is the sphere of wisdom— both the wisdom of the heart and the wisdom of the mind. Imagine that in this heaven you see two rings of dancing lights, one ring within the other, each reflecting the other, and moving in twin circles. The lights move as beautifully as two concentrically moving rainbows or a moving double garland of flowers.

Realize that in true wisdom the mind and heart are not at odds with each other but rather move joyfully and harmoniously together. Imagine what it would feel like if your mind and heart were coordinated in their wisdom and their purpose, and let this sense of intellectual and emotional integration fill your body. Enjoy the experience of being wise in heart and mind and having heart and mind in perfect alignment with each other. Then when you feel ready, ascend with your guide to the next sphere, the Heaven of Mars.

THE HEAVEN OF MARS—DEDICATION & COURAGE

The Heaven of Mars is the sphere of dedication to a higher purpose and the courage that this dedication entails. Imagine that in this sphere of Paradise you see a red star whose rays gently warm and support you. As you bask in these gentle rays, dedicate yourself to fulfilling your Divine mission of helping make the earth a paradise.

Give thanks to all your ancestors for being the conduits for your entry into the physical world, and wish the best for all your descendants, whether in this, future, or previous lifetimes. Let a sense of dedication and courageous commitment fill your entire body. After you have thoroughly experienced this sense of renewed purpose, ascend with your guide to the next level of Paradise, the Heaven of Jupiter.

THE HEAVEN OF JUPITER—PEACE AND ORDER

The Heaven of Jupiter is the realm of peace on earth and the establishment of Divine order in the lives of all nations. Justice is the theme of this level of Paradise, as it was in the Heaven of Mercury, but the focus is on the long-term end results or fruits of justice rather than on justice as the restorative process.

In this heaven, imagine that you see an enormous eagle, a classical symbol of just government. The eagle is brilliantly luminous, and on closer inspection you realize that the eagle's body is not solid but rather consists of numerous points of light, or luminous souls, arranging themselves in the shape of an eagle.

Become aware that peace on earth, security, and justice for all people depend on the cooperation of all of us and on our willingness to act from the level of the Soul rather than the level of purely personal self-interest. As you watch the shining eagle, affirm that peace on earth is prevailing.

Imagine how you would feel if you received word that combatants in some major trouble spot had decided to make peace and forgive each other, and let a sense of wonder and relief flow through you. After you have enjoyed this experience, ascend with your guide to the seventh level of Paradise, the Heaven of Saturn.

THE HEAVEN OF SATURN—CONTEMPLATION

The Heaven of Saturn is the sphere of contemplation, or meditation on the Divine. In this level of Paradise, imagine that you see a golden ladder that is so high that its top is beyond your field of vision. See many individual flames of light descending the ladder. The golden ladder symbolizes the connecting pathway between our daily lives and the Divine that contemplation affords us. The descending lights symbolize the descent of Divine qualities into our lives when we ascend in consciousness to the Divine in our meditation practice.

Observe the descending lights closely, and become aware of the loving-kindness emanating from them. Imagine that the descending flames of light are bringing Divine grace and mercy into all aspects of your life. Feel deep gratitude, and let gratitude fill every part of your body. Then when you feel ready, soar with your guide up the golden ladder and into the Heaven of the Fixed Stars.

THE HEAVEN OF THE FIXED STARS—
FAITH, HOPE, AND CHARITY

The Heaven of the Fixed Stars is the realm of faith, hope, and charity. Standing in the Heaven of the Fixed Stars, look down at the seven previous heavens and the Earth below them. See how Divine Light is flowing down and permeating them. Then notice three bright lights shining before you in the Heaven of the Fixed Stars. These lights represent great masters of faith, hope, and charity, respectively.

Approach the first light and bask in its rays. Realize that this light is strengthening your faith in the goodness of life and your link with the Divine. Be filled with a sense of increased faith. Approach the second light, and similarly let its rays gently warm you. Realize that this light is strengthening your hope for a better world. Be filled with a new sense of expectation that things are changing for the better and that our mission of creating Paradise on Earth is being fulfilled.

Finally, approach the third light and let its gentle warmth suffuse you. Realize that this light is strengthening you in charity, or love of neighbor. Be filled with increased compassion for others and an increased desire to alleviate their suffering. Then when you are ready, rise with your guide to the next sphere of Paradise, the Primum Mobile.

THE PRIMUM MOBILE—UNMOVED MOVER

In the medieval mind, the Primum Mobile (Latin for "first mover") is that sphere which is itself unmoved but which moves all others below it by directing the light of God down to them from the level above it, known as the Empyrean. The Primum Mobile is the realm of angels.

After you rise with your guide to the Primum Mobile, once again look down and see the levels below you (the Heaven of the Fixed Stars, the seven planetary Heavens, and finally the Earth), all filled with Divine Light. Really feel the connection between the Earth and the higher levels of Paradise.

Then in the Primum Mobile see before you in the distance a point of light far more intense than anything you have seen so far. This is the point of Divine Light which reflects down from the Empyrean and which represents God's love as it sustains the entire universe.

Around this point of light see nine concentric circles of angels dancing. Each circle contains that order of angels responsible for one of the nine spheres we have visited, with the Seraphim, the order who are custodians of the Primum Mobile, being closest to the point of light and circling the fastest.

As you observe the dancing circles of angels, unite your purpose with that of the angels in diffusing Divine Light throughout the universe. Realize that in creating Paradise on Earth, you are fulfilling your mandate as the angels fulfill theirs. Watch this vision of dancing angels until it slowly fades away.

THE EMPYREAN—MAXIMUM CONTACT WITH THE DIVINE

When the vision has faded away, realize that without doing anything overt, you and your guide have entered into the highest level of Paradise, the heaven of pure light known as the Empyrean. This is the place of our maximum contact with the Divine, which Itself is above even the Empyrean.

In the Empyrean, see flowing before you a river of pure golden light whose two banks are covered with beautiful flowers. Living sparks fly out of the flowers and back into the river again, in a constant flow of coming and going. As you gaze at this remarkable sight, the scene transforms itself. The river has become a massive white rose of incredible, luminous beauty.

Dwelling in the petals of the white rose are all those blessed souls who have achieved union with the Divine and thus experience eternal bliss. As you gaze at this magnificent sight, feel that there is a place for you, too, in this rose. Experience yourself dwelling within it. Feel that you have returned home to your loving Source and let deep inner peace and trust flow through every cell of your body. Feel completely loved and cherished by the Divine.

After you have enjoyed this experience for as long as you like, imagine that you are raising your eyes in the Empyrean up towards the Eternal Light. Mentally express your gratitude for this experience and state your wish that all beings may attain the bliss of Paradise.

RETURN TO EVERYDAY REALITY

Then prepare to return to everyday reality. Remain with your eyes still closed as you slowly return to normal consciousness. After you return to normal consciousness, keep your eyes closed and spend at least a couple of minutes thinking about the soles of your feet, so that your energy will be appropriately grounded. Then very slowly open your eyes.

This visualization does not take very long to perform, although the above account of it may seem a bit lengthy.

If there is a certain part of the visualization that seems especially meaningful to you, feel free to work with that section alone or even to adapt its use in ways that are appropriate for you. For example, one man whom I acquainted with this visualization felt that he lacked charity and wanted to increase his tolerance of the people around him at his office. He decided to work every day for a week with the Heaven of the Fixed Stars visualization, in which he could receive the rays of the light that would increase his love of neighbor.

Another friend decided that she would concentrate on the Heaven of Venus visualization to put herself in the right mindset for finding a husband. Her adaptation consisted of prefacing the visualization by reading through a list of the qualities she wanted in a mate, such as generosity, sexual compatibility, etc. She would then go the Heaven of Venus in visualization to see a symbol of love, feel intense love for her unknown future husband, and express appreciation for all his good qualities.

Though I myself enjoy doing the entire visualization, I frequently use just the White Rose section to quickly renew myself, always visualizing myself as healthy, beautiful, and trim as I receive love from the White Rose.

If working with a single section, you can see yourself ascending quickly with your guide through the various levels of Paradise until you reach your desired level, or you can simply see yourself with your guide already in the desired level. In either case, it is a good idea to ground yourself after you finish the visualization by thinking about your feet before you open your eyes.

Once a friend with a particularly strong capacity for visualization told me that she felt dizzy from ascending through the levels of Paradise, as though she had actually gone up into very high altitudes! This is a rare reaction, but in case you should feel dizzy or feel pressure in your head when doing the visualization, you can alter the vertical format. You can think of each new level as representing a change in focus, and you can imagine yourself and your guide as switching focus from one Heaven to the next, much like switching to a different TV channel, rather than as ascending.

When you can, do take time to perform the entire visualization. People who perform it have reported increased experiences of joy and a strengthening of their conviction that the goal of our sojourn on Earth is to mirror here the love, harmony, artistry, and beauty of Paradise.

"IMPARADISE" YOURSELF!

I hope that you have enjoyed reading this book, and I feel confident that the suggestions given in this chapter and the previous chapters will be useful to you. The final page of this book—"When Facing Temptation"—gives a list of selected things to do when facing temptation that you can photocopy, carry with you, and consult as needed.

If I could sum up the message of this book in one sentence, it would be "Don't imprison yourself; *imparadise yourself!*" *Imparadise* is a word made up by Dante that we can use as our motto in creating a better life for ourselves and others. Imparadise yourself now! I know that you can do it. I'm wishing you the very best in reaching your perfect weight—and in every other aspect of your great work of creating Paradise on Earth!

WHEN FACING TEMPTATION

Copy this page and carry it with you to consult as needed.

ASK YOURSELF

1. *Am I really hungry, or am I nervous?*
2. *Would I rather eat this or be thin?*
3. *Is there enough life force in this food
   to be worth the calories?*

TELL YOURSELF

1. *Faster to my goal!*
2. *Food is not love.*
3 *Other people can resist this, and so can I.*
4. *I only have to resist a few times for it to be easy.*

INSTEAD OF EATING YOU CAN

1. *Remember your goal weight.*
2. *Articulate your feelings.*
3. *Look at your hands.*
4. *Take deep breaths.*
5. *Breathe purple air.*
6. *Have a mind snack.*
7. *Pray for help.*
8. *Leave the scene.*
9. *Consider a substitute.*
10. *Postpone gratification.*